CANCER

Why what you don't know about your treatment could harm you.

Holly Fourchalk, Ph.D., DNM®, RHT, HT

CHOICES UNLIMITED
FOR
HEALTH & WELLNESS

CANCER

Cancer **DOES NOT** have to be a
death sentence.

Cancer **DOES NOT** have to be a prolonged
journey through hell.

Cancer **IS** a symptom to work with. Learn
to engage your body's natural healing
mechanisms.

Holly Fourchalk, PhD., DNM®, RHT, HT

CHOICES UNLIMITED
FOR
HEALTH **&** WELLNESS

Dr. Holly Fourchalk, Ph.D., DNM®, RHT, HT
Tel: 604.764.5203
Fax: 604.465.7964
Website: www.choicesunlimited.ca
E-mail: holly@choicesunlimited.ca

Editing, Interior Design and Cover Design:
Wendy Dewar Hughes, Summer Bay Press

ISBN: 978-1-927626-08-5
Digital ISBN: 978-1-927626-09-2

This book includes neither an exhaustive nor exclusive list of alternative options for working with cancer.

Rather, it provides an overview of theories, foods, herbs and modalities with which the patient or practitioner may work.

My company is called Choices Unlimited for Health and Wellness for a reason. There is a wide number of choices to choose from with regard to maximizing your health. We can only make good, effective choices when we have a working knowledge of what those choices may be.

If a given modality or protocol resonates for you, research it further. Explore your options within the profile. Your mind is a very powerful tool – make it work for you. Regardless of what you choose to do, make the placebo effect – or the power of the mind – be a part of your healing journey.

Here's to your journey into health.

DISCLAIMER

Every effort has been made by the author to ensure that the information in this book is as accurate as possible. However, it is by no means a complete or exhaustive examination of all information.

The author knows what worked for her and what has worked for others but no two people are the same and so the author cannot and does not render judgment or advice regarding a particular individual.

Further, because our bodies are unique any two individuals may experience different results from the same therapy.

The author believes in both prevention and the superiority of a natural non-invasive approach over drugs and surgery.

The information herein is presented by yet another researcher, whose sources come from around the world and has been accumulated over the past 30 years.

Research has shown that one of the top three leading causes of death in North America occurs because of the physician/pharmaceutical component of the scenario.

Perhaps the real leading cause of death and disability is a result of the lack of awareness of natural therapies. These therapies are well known to prevent and treat many common degenerative, inflammatory and oxidative diseases.

The author loves to research and loves to teach. This book is another attempt to increase awareness about health and the many options we have to bring the body back into a healthy balance.

Ever-increasing numbers of people are aware of healing foods and herbs, supplements and modalities but there are still far too many who are not. The fact that our physicians are part of this latter group makes healing even more challenging.

The unfortunate fact is, those who can profit from sickness and disease promote ignorance and the results are devastating.

It is not the intent of the author that anyone should choose to read this book and make decisions regarding their health or medical care based on ideas contained in this book.

Rather, the intent is to provide an overview of the cancer industry and various alternative understandings of the evolution of cancer and the various types of healing processes to engage in. Beyond that, it is the responsibility of the individual to find a health care practitioner to work with to achieve optimal health.

The author and publisher are not responsible for any adverse effects or consequences resulting from the use of any of the suggestions or information contained in the book but offer this material as information that the public has a right to hear and utilize at its own discretion.

To my Parents

For all their support and encouragement
My Dad for his ever-listening ear
My mother for her open mind

CANCER

CONTENTS

ONE

Introduction

"Cancer" has been turned into something worse than a four-letter word, yet, it shouldn't be.

I had an ovarian tumor over thirty years ago. I was told on a Friday afternoon that I needed surgery immediately Monday morning.

After coming out of shock, I phoned my osteopath-naturopath who put me on a simple diet. The tumor was gone in three and a half weeks!

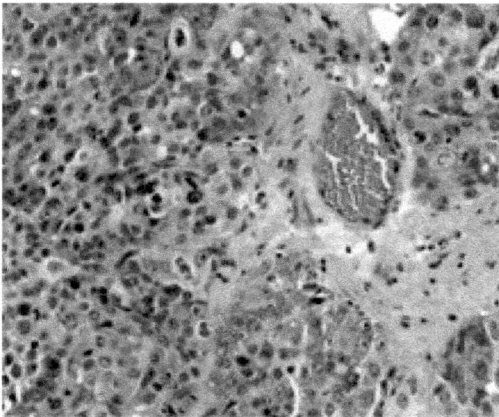

(Ovarian cancer)

Unfortunately, a great deal of peer-reviewed information published in "scientific journals" is not scientific. In today's world, the content in those publications is often bought and paid for.

Real researchers know that, balk at it and criticize mainstream journals. They know that if their work goes against pharmaceutical companies (and their profits), their work simply won't get published in these journals.

Pharmaceutical companies have been known to alter, modify and eliminate data so that they obtain their patents. Doctors can be paid to market and recommend pharmaceuticals. Doctors can also be paid huge amounts of money to run clients through studies in their offices.

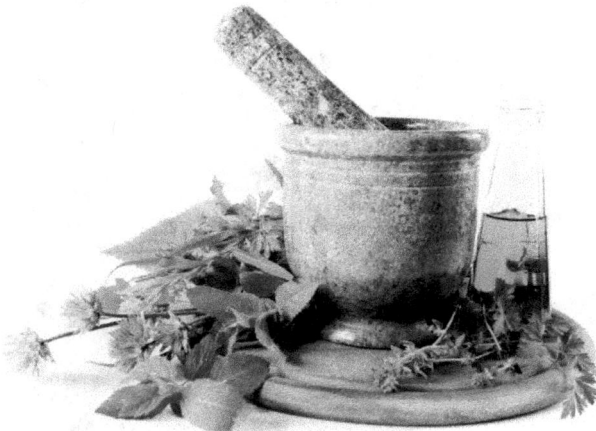

Natural or alternative therapies are considered unscientific by mainstream medicine whereas inorganic, man-made, artificial, synthetic chemicals are somehow considered more powerful and effective than real live food, nutrients and molecules.

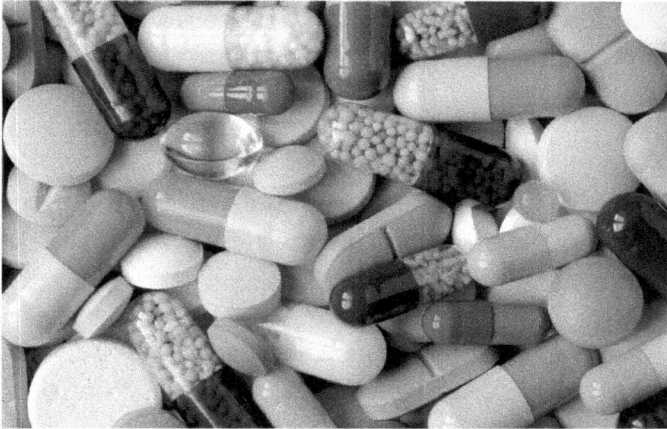

Our bodies utilize the nutrients in foods and herbs to make over 10,000 enzymes, over 100 hormones, over 50 neurotransmitters, over 30 types of collagens and more. When you consider that our real food is not only depleted in nutrients but that we are eating artificial, processed, microwaved, fast "food" that has no nutrient quality, isn't it a logical assumption that our bodies may depleted in nutrition?

The wisdom of the body is still far beyond our current understanding and we are still struggling to figure out how the body functions. Perhaps we should utilize the body to heal itself. After all, that is what it was designed to do.

Where did we come up with such narcissistic arrogance as to say that man could make a dead, artificial, synthetic product in the laboratory and it would be better than what we find in nature?

Repeatedly, the evidence shows us that the more man gets involved with anything from the food we eat to the medicine we take, the more toxic it becomes.

Most natural therapies are actually very inexpensive, safe and effective but you have to do the research and take responsibility for your health.

Even the health care system knows that they can't make health happen. Trained to manage symptoms, not health, MDs are not taught about health or functional medicine. They are taught about sickness and how to manage it. That, of course, supports the pharmaceutical companies.

So let's learn about health, vitality and harmony in the body. After all, if we understand it then maybe we can manage it.

TWO

Healthy Cells

What is a healthy cell?

Do you want to become a cellular biologist, a geneticist or a biochemist? Probably not. If you did, you would probably be in school with the old outdated textbooks.

Perhaps you are looking at what an unhealthy nation we have and want to protect your health.

We are going simplify the subject of what a healthy cell is but first, let me tell you where I am coming from. Before I became a Doctor of Natural Medicine, I ran a clinic as a Registered Psychologist for some twenty years. I learned that often those struggling were simply victims of their environments. I also learned that many victims of physical and psychological problems created their own destructive environments. So the task at hand was often how to change a "victim" into a "survivor". From there we need to determine how to change a "survivor" into a "thriver".

I look at our health in much the same way. Some processes, cells, organs and systems become a victim to their environment and some will create a victimized environment.

Let's begin with the healthy cell. It should be full of life with over thirteen different types of organelles (cell organs) in it. The brain of the cell is not the nucleus as man historically thought but rather the gonads. Every cell in the body has all the systems that the entire body has...so the reproductive system in the human, are the gonads; but the reproductive system of the cell is called the nucleus. Likewise, the organizational system of the body is the brain, but the organizational system of the cell is the membrane.

Today it is recognized that the membrane around the cell also acts as the brain. The membrane decides what needs to go into the cell and what needs to be eliminated from the cell. The function of the membrane itself is a very complicated process with various different types of transport and diffusion processes and an awful lot of coming and going.

Inside the cell we have an enormous number of processes going on creating energy to fuel the processes, such as, creating (anabolic) enzymes, hormones, neurotransmitters, transport mechanisms, DNA, mRNA, detoxing, replicating, communicating, digesting and breaking down (catabolic). As in the whole body, so does the individual cell.

Cancer cells have one major difference from other cells. Their apoptosis is turned off. What does this mean? Apoptosis is automatic, pre-programmed death. If that is turned off then the cell keeps replicating and replicating without ever dying.

Most chemo/radio therapies therefore focus on killing off these rapidly replicating cells that utilize all our nutrients. But other cells also replicate fast and we do not set out to kill them at cost to the whole. So why do we do this with cancer cells?

The problem is that the conventional therapies typically cause more harm than health and are costly to the pocketbook as well. Typically, the life experience engaged in while going through the toxic process is also horrific. Furthermore, the success rate is dismal. So, besides the pharmaceutical companies, who actually benefits?

THREE

Different theories on the evolution of cancer

Let's now explore a few different theories and research outcomes regarding the evolution of cancer and its treatment.

First, it is important to realize that most cancers can take a long time to evolve to the point of detection. Likewise, once the cancer is theoretically removed, patients are considered cured only after cancer has not been detected for five years. (Unfortunately, a patient could die of cancer the day following detection and it wouldn't change the way the stats are calculated.)

Rife

A researcher called Rife was a very interesting man and had a very different perspective on the subject of cancer than his peers had. He discovered that pathogens change. They grow and develop into many different forms not unlike how a caterpillar metamorphoses into a butterfly. Rife discovered that fungus and yeast change into bacteria which can then further change into a virus.

In support of this kind of research, one doctor claimed that he never seen a cancer patient who did not also have a yeast infection (Candida).

Rife - pathogens

Rife found that when he injected rats with a virus that caused them to develop cancer he was also able to eliminate the virus by treating them with a specific radio frequency which eliminated the cancer. In this case, what he found was that the virus' protein coating allowed it to bond to a healthy cell membrane and thus get inside the cell. The virus would then, in effect, steal the DNA of the mitochondria inside the cell. (The mitochondria are organelles that amongst other things, produce the fuel for the cell, called Adenosine Triphosphate or ATP.) If the virus could access the ATP it had the energy it required to keep going. The virus would replicate, access more and more of the mitochondria and simply keep growing. (Note: a given cell will have many mitochondria depending on the amount of energy the given cell requires. Therefore, a heart cell will have in excess of a 1000 mitochondria.).

Unfortunately, the virus also produces toxins.

Between the "stolen energy" and the "increased toxicity" the cell loses its capacity to metabolize oxygen. The cell becomes anaerobic, utilizing fermentation to create energy, which is far more ineffective and produces less energy what it should normally be doing.

If this happens to a cell, the cell has become a victim to the virus. To kill all the subsequent cancer cells would be highly toxic to the body and would need an extremely healthy liver to eliminate all the toxic damage.

The challenge with some of these pathogens that can invade a cell and leave toxins behind is that they have a protein coating that surrounds the cell and keeps it hidden from the immune system, something like a "cloaking device" in Star Wars movies that keeps the ship hidden from sight.

But how did this start in the first place? Can a pathogen just take up residence wherever it wants or does it require a given environment in order to live and replicate?

Apoptosis

Another explanation for the development of cancer cells is that they got "screwed up" in the replicating process. The apoptosis got turned off and there wasn't anybody around at the

time to either correct the faulty DNA or eliminate the new disorganized cell. Apoptosis is
preprogrammed cell death.

So how come there wasn't sufficient clean-up
crew around to either re-structure the DNA
before the new cell took off or kill it before it
left camp?

pH

Some claim that cancer is a result of a poor pH
level in the body. While the pH can be as low
as 1.8 in the stomach and as high as 8.1 in the
pancreatic secretions, each component of the
body requires a different pH level in order for
the enzymes in that area to function effectively.
In addition, it is believed that cancer cells alter
their own pH levels by taking in glucose (very
acidic) and preventing oxygen (alkaline).

In our society, we have a very acidic diet which
would enable the pathogens that thrive in an
acidic environment to take over from those
that thrive in a more alkaline environment.

Our bodies are designed with a number of
ways to maintain healthy pH levels but over
time, these can fail and that is when imbalance
leads to dysfunction and disease. We have both
short term and long-term ways of managing
our pH levels:

Short term:

Body flushes out acidic waste through the respiratory system (breathing in oxygen and breathing out carbon dioxide) and the kidney system

Long term:

If, over time, chronically low pH levels are endured, the body will work with secondary methods releasing alkalizing minerals from the body:
- Calcium from the bones and teeth
- Magnesium from our blood vessels
- Potassium from our neuromuscular system
- Sodium from our joints

If we do not correct our pH balance, enzymes stop functioning and the body starts to break down.

Anti-oxidants

Others will claim that it is the lack of anti-oxidants in the body that cause cancers, in particular, a glutathione deficiency. Why glutathione? Well, because it is the master anti-oxidant. It is the only anti-oxidant that can re-cycle itself and it can also re-cycle all the other anti-oxidants.

In addition, it is involved in so many other functions throughout the body. While there are in excess of 40,000 articles on Vitamin C on the Pubmed.com website and more than 49,000 articles on Vitamin D, there are over 95,000 articles on glutathione.

Yet, most physicians I talk with don't even remember learning about it from their schooling days, never mind have any idea of the immense amount of research done on glutathione in the last ten years alone.

Because we have so much adrenal, high-stress functioning in our systems; such an immense amount of herbicides, pesticides, and other toxic chemicals in our foods; such a huge number of toxic, artificial, synthetic drugs that are prescribed and so little actual nutrition, our bodies are depleted of good anti-oxidants and full of free radicals.

The free radicals further destroy our bodies and provide a chemical dump for pathogens to grow in. And thus, we end up with cancer.

German New Medicine

German New Medicine is a protocol that began

with a physician/scientist called Ryke Geer Hamer. Dr. Hamer claimed that all cancers began in the mind. He did extensive research identifying which kind of psychological traumas resulted in what kinds of cancer.

He claimed that how we interpret and respond to the world with respect to repeated trauma, especially when it is repressed, determines whether or not we are likely to end up with cancers. He also believed that cancers can be hugely dealt with and effectively if we follow the protocol. The father of German New Medicine was apparently taken to court in Germany and despite having to show his files, which revealed a 98% success rate, he lost his position in the hospital and in the university.
However, there are people around the world, both allopathic and otherwise that follow his teachings.

It is rather strange that arguments against revolve around the fact that he was not able to cure everyone...yet conventional treatments have far less effectiveness than he had – and they are allowed to continue...

He claims that there are 5 rules biological rules:

- 1st law ("Iron Rule"): Severe diseases originate from a shock event, which is experienced by the individual as very difficult, highly acute, dramatic and isolating. The shock's psychological conflict content determines the location of the appearance of a focus of activity in the brain that can be seen in a CT scan as a set of concentric rings, called "Hamer foci," which correspond to the location of the disease in the body. The subsequent development of the conflict determines the development of both the brain focus and the disease.

- 2nd law (Two phased nature of disease): A patient who has not solved their conflict is in the first, active conflict phase, where the sympathetic nervous system dominates and which manifests as a "cold disease" accompanied by cold skin and extremities, stress, weight loss and sleep disorders. If they manage to resolve the conflict, they enter a second, post-resolution healing phase, in which the parasympathetic nervous system, commonly diagnosed as a separate "warm" (Rheumatic, infectious, allergic, etc) disease. This second phase is the one that usually entails more risks, and a complete cure only comes upon its completion. In some circumstances, not solving the conflict but downgrading it to a reasonably livable level may be preferable than facing the second phase.

- 3rd law (Ontogenetic system of diseases): Hamer proposes that disease progression is primarily controlled by the brain, either by the "old brain" (brain stem and cerebellum) or the "new brain" (cerebrum). The old brain controls more primitive processes, having to do with basic survival, such as breathing, eating, and reproduction, whereas the new brain manages more advanced personal and social issues, such as territorial conflicts, separation conflicts and self-devaluation and identity conflicts. Hamer's research is tied to the science of embryology because he links the type of disease progression — whether involving tissue augmentation (tumor growth), tissue loss (necrosis or ulceration) or functional impairment — with the embryonic germ layer (endoderm, mesoderm or ectoderm) from which both the organ tissues and the corresponding brain regions originate. Conflicts which have their focus either in the brain stem (which controls body tissues that derive from the endoderm) or the cerebellum (which controls tissues that derive from the mesoderm) show cell multiplication in the conflict active phase, and destruction of the resulting tumors in the healing phase. Cerebrum directed conflicts (affecting the rest of mesoderm-derived tissues and all ectoderm-derived ones) show either cell decrease (necrosis, ulcers) or function impairment or interruption in the active phase, and the replenishment of the damaged tissues in the healing phase (which can also be diagnosed as a tumor).

- 4th law (Ontogenetic system of microbes): Microbes do not cause diseases but are used by the body, coordinated by the brain, to optimize the healing phase, provided that the required microbes are available when needed. Fungi and mycobacteria work on tissues that originated in the endoderm, as well as on some of the tissues originating in the mesoderm. Bacteria work on all mesoderm derived tissues and viruses on ectoderm derived ones. Hamer maintains that these microbes, rather than being antagonistic to the body, actually perform a necessary role in healing. And that some of the interventions of conventional medicine are counterproductive, by interfering with these natural processes.

- 5th law ("Quintessence"): The conflict active phase and the healing phase of diseases, as described above, constitute "special meaningful programs of nature," developed during the evolution of the species, to allow organisms to override everyday functioning in order to deal with particular emergency situations.

Source:
http://en.wikipedia.org/wiki/German_New_Medicine

When one studies the healing modality and the research behind it, one finds a lot of controversial arguments. It is interesting that the pharmaceutical / medical organizations struggle to prove that it is wrong rather than coming from a purely scientific perspective and looking to see if there is a truth in the hypothesis.

FOUR

Diagnostic tools for cancer

There are a lot of tools out there to diagnose cancer but are they ineffective. There is also a lot of controversy over the use of various diagnostic tools. Let's look at some of it.

The Prostate Specific Antigen (PSA) tests and mammograms are probably two of the most controversial diagnostic protocols in use today. In fact, in recent times it looks like both are being "phased out" as their lack of usefulness is recognized.

PSA

PSAs are utilized to determine if there are cancerous issues with the prostate and, as a man ages, the use of this test has been promoted on a more regular basis. The older a man got the more often he was told he had to have the test. But the use of the PSA test to test for prostate cancer is finally on its way out.

The U.S. Preventive Services Task Force has formally given a "D" grade to the PSA test. That is the lowest possible grade the agency issues. What it means is that the risks of the test outweigh the benefits.

See:
http://general-medicine.jwatch.org › Specialties › General Medicine

www.medpagetoday.com/MeetingCoverage/AUA/32817

Many physicians want to keep using the PSA along with men who believe the test led to a prostate surgery that saved their lives but there is a big challenge.

In reality, the new studies are pretty consistent – so consistent that I don't understand why this new recommendation is controversial.

As it turns out, the PSA test has an incredibly high rate of false positives – as high as 80 percent. You might want to accept that the high level if it actually saved lives the other 20 percent of the time but that is not the case.

Instead, the PSA usually leads to treatments such as medications and surgery that can come with serious long-term risks like incontinence and impotence. Studies are now revealing that the medications for an enlarged prostate may actually cause prostate cancer – not a good trade off. Further, other studies are showing that men survive quite well without any of the treatments that cause such devastating side effects.

Why? Evidently, prostate tumors grow very slowly and most patients will live quite well with them and if it hadn't been for the PSA, would never have even known that they had them and would certainly not die from them.

This is the reason that the USPSTF is abandoning the test. This is also the reason that many wise physicians stopped using the PSA a long time ago. It is also the reason that Dr. Richard Ablin, who identified the test, regretted it.

Ablin's op-ed two years ago noted that 30 million American men were getting the test every year at a cost of $3 billion, much of it paid by Medicare and the Veteran's Administration. "The test's popularity," he wrote, "has led to a hugely expensive public health disaster." Unfortunately, the PSA – has been costly both financially (to the Medicare system and the personal pocket) and psychologically (for all those who were falsely identified). It has also been physically challenging for those who were prescribed drugs and or surgery thanks to false diagnoses from the PSA.

http://reforminghealth.org/2012/04/25/on-prostate-cancer-screening-warren-buffet-and-ignoring-science/

Mammogram

Mammogram is another test that is being phased out of the system. Not long ago, the mammogram was pushed on a regular basis by many physicians and still is.

Why is it now being eliminated?

Reports vary but most reports claim that false positives on mammograms range around 89% and the new research shows that these false positives have a 67% higher risk factor of developing cancer.

http://www.naturalnews.com/022227.html
http://abcnews.go.com/Health/CancerPreve
ntionAndTreatment/breast-cancer-women-
false-positive-mammograms-higher-
risk/story?id=16078223

Today, it is also recognized that if a woman has a mammogram for ten years in a row, she will accumulate the same amount of radiation as if she had been standing a mile away from Nagasaki or Hiroshima when the atomic bombs went off.

In Dr. Frank Shallenberger's newsletter (February 2010), he writes, "Many so-called experts claim mammograms have saved millions of lives. They always cite the fact that breast cancer rates have come down significantly in recent years...The truth of the matter is that breast cancer rates have come down because women stopped using synthetic hormone replacement therapy."

(RHT - replacement hormone therapy is an issue that will be dealt with in another book. It is yet another pharmaceutical ploy that harmed far too many women.)

Another reason for the phasing out of mammograms is that researchers have discovered that radiation exposure can alter the cells' microenvironment. Altering the surrounding environment greatly raises the odds that future cells will become cancerous, according to Researchers at the U.S. Department of Energy's Lawrence Berkeley National Laboratory (Berkeley Lab).

"...by getting normal cells to prematurely age and stop dividing, the radiation exposure created space for epigenetically altered cells that would otherwise have been filled by normal cells. In other words, the radiation promoted the growth of pre-cancerous cells by making the environment that surrounded the cells more hospitable to their continued growth," says Paul Yaswen, a cell biologist and breast cancer research specialist with Berkeley Lab's Life Sciences Division, said in a statement to the press.

Learn more:
http://www.naturalnews.com/028959_radiati on_brst_cancer.html#ixzz2EJykLnyX

http://newscenter.lbl.gov/news-releases/2010/05/13/new-concerns-about-radiation-and-breast-cancer/

http://www.cancer-health.info/new-concerns-about-radiation-and-breast-cancer-raised-in-study/

This is not good, no matter how you look at it. Further, the researchers acknowledged that the levels of radiation that they used in their exper-iments were not as much as a single exposure through a routine mammogram but rather comparable to that received through a CT scan or radiotherapy, which of course, raises a whole other conglomerate of questions.

In addition, like the PSA, the false positives and false negatives are very high. Moreover, mammograms compress the breasts so tightly that if there was cancer growth the compres-sion could lead to a lethal spread of cancerous cells.

Research shows that now that the mammograms are not being pushed, not only are breast cancers lower but so are other cancer statistics.

"Otis Brawley, the Chief Medical Officer of the American Cancer Society, made a stunning and controversial announcement that we are over-screening for breast and prostate cancer, that results in a large number of people being treated for cancer when it really isn't needed. Screening the healthy population, results in identifying and treating a large number of false positives, and tumors that will never actually become cancerous. He also states that the American Cancer Society may have exaggerated the health benefits of screening. (ABC Nightly News)"

See:
http://www.holistichelp.net/blog/8-reasons-you-shouldnt-have-a-mammogram/

In addition, the US Preventative Services Task Force is stirring up controversy suggesting that women in their forties should NOT get routine mammograms.

The following statement about mammograms was made in the Lancet in July of 1995: "The benefit is marginal, the harm caused is substantial, and the costs incurred are enormous..."

Dr. Mercola made the following statement. "Women have unnecessarily undergone mastectomies, radiation and chemotherapy after receiving false positives on a mammogram.

See:
http://articles.mercola.com/sites/articles/arc
hive/2009/12/05/Avoid-Routine-
Mammograms-if-You-are-Under-50.aspx

But now look what we have! 3-D mammograms. Dr. Douglass has a website called www.healthiertalk.com and he claims that this new 3-D mammogram does improve accuracy by 7% but it emits twice the radiation of the traditional screening. So even if you didn't have cancer prior to your mammogram – you might have it afterwards!

See:
http://www.healthiertalk.com/3-d-
mammograms-present-new-risks-women-3500

The challenge is with women whose lives were saved because of a mammograms and subsequent biopsies – what do we say to them? Well, there are a few detection devices at present that don't appear to have all the massive concerns.

1. Thermographic screening measures radiation of infrared heat from your body and translates it into anatomical images. There is no use of ionizing radiation and apparently the screening can detect breast cancer ten years earlier than either a physical exam or a mammography. It does this with the detection of angiogenesis – or new blood vessels – which tumors have to create before they can reach any appreciable size.

2. There are various devices such as photon resonance that can provide information on thousands of variables within the body, thus telling where the imbalance is and how to correct it. The wonderful aspect of something that works on photon resonance is that it is providing treatment while accumulating the information.

In addition, we also have to acknowledge that other diagnostic tools can cause cancer as well not just the ones used to detect cancer.

For instance, according to two studies done on CT scans performed in 2007, these scans caused 29,000 cancers and killed nearly 15,000 Americans. Unfortunately, we don't know how many of the patients may have already had undetected growing cancers but what they did know was that about 70 million CT scans were done on Americans in 2007, up from 3 million in 1980.

See:
http://www.pbs.org/newshour/rundown/20
09/12/study-ct-scan-overuse-could-lead-to-
cancer-deaths.html

Further, that doesn't tell us the percentage per
population, as there was obviously a population growth during that time as well. However,
it is pretty safe to say that there was huge a
profit made at the cost of a lot of lives.

See:
http://www.msnbc.msn.com/id/34420356/

References:
http://www.naturalnews.com/028959_radiati
on_brst_cancer.html#ixzz1zL6iwmDA

http://www.naturalnews.com/028959_radiati
on_brst_cancer.html#ixzz1zL8YQJNt

http://www.ncbi.nlm.nih.gov/pubmed/20146
798

http://envirocancer.cornell.edu/factsheet/ph
ysical/fs52.radiation.cfm...

FIVE

When you get the diagnosis – what happens?

I can remember, having gone through blood tests and ultrasounds and everything else I did thirty years ago when I was diagnosed with cancer.

I was sitting in one of those little white cloaks you used to have to wear when you went into see the doctor, in this tiny little cubicle and waiting, without much concern. Then this little tiny female physician waltzed in. Nothing to be concerned about, I thought, except she said, "You know that ball you saw on the ultrasound? Well, it is a tumor and it is dangerous and fatal. We need you to make an appointment for first thing Monday morning to have surgery and we will take it out."

She looked for agreement and then walked out. That was it. She left and I sat there. And sat there. And sat there. I had seen many people die of cancer already in my life. This was not good news.

I have no idea how long it was before I was

able to pull myself together and get dressed and leave the little room.

I know I did not make any arrangements for surgery Monday morning. My husband honked at me as I roamed aimlessly around the parking lot looking for our car. He asked if I had seen a ghost. I replied that I hadn't but explained what the doctor said.

Now it was his turn. He went into shock, and the two of us sat there not knowing what to do. When you get the diagnoses of cancer, there is immediate fear and shock. The oncologist is the trained specialist and so he or she has the upper hand. You may or may not be forewarned of the following:

- What the short term and long term side effects are
- What the real evidence says
- What the costs are and more.

There is a high probability that you won't be told about:

1. What the alternative options are
2. Where to go for alternative therapies
3. What the real evidence says about these therapies.

The reasons you won't be told:

- The doctor doesn't want to lose that paycheck.

- He doesn't know.

- He or she is not a cancer therapist, rather a chemotherapist specialist.

- She has been told and read that alternative therapies are ineffective. After all, articles about them are not even allowed in mainstream journals. Even Western allopathic scientists cannot get their articles published if they negate Western pharmaceuticals so your doctor must really want to learn about other ways to help you heal.

- He has no background in nutritional and herbal training. (Typically, a medical doctor receives only three and half hours of nutrition instruction in over four years of schooling.)

- He has no background in homeopathies, Ayurvedic or Traditional Chinese Medicine or any other modality.

- She is trained in Western synthetic, artificial, man- made drugs and is only registered to prescribe these.

The oncologist has been taught that "modern" medicine has the answers and he is only trained in how to prescribe these artificial, synthetic, man-made chemicals that are toxic to the body.

You may have noticed that I feel strongly about his problem. Now you know a little about why that is.

Remember, if it is natural, pharmaceutical companies cannot patent it or make money from it. This is one reason we are now seeing a trend emerge where pharmaceutical companies are buying out nutriceutical companies. It is also why Big Pharma wants to control supplements. The more people look towards natural remedies, the more natural remedies become a profit resource. So now there is an increasing amount of money to be made there.

The challenge is that, you, the patient, have no training in any of the modalities. You were taught to go to the "doctor" and he will make you better. You do not have a PhD in research and design, degrees in genetics, cellular biology, organic chemistry, etc. So you rely on what your expert "sickness management specialist" tells you.

SIX

Do the conventional treatments work?

In conventional medicine, we have a variety of options:

- different types of chemotherapy
- different types of radiation
- surgery

Did you know that upwards of 90% of oncologists would not take chemo or radiation therapy themselves? (Differing results depend on the particular study.)

That doesn't sound so good to me. This situation is similar to war. If the government officials who want to declare war had to send their own children first, there might be no war. They would probably find different strategies, likewise with cancer. If the oncologist who is willing to prescribe chemotherapy had to have gone through a bout of chemotherapy first, I am sure the strategy might change.

(Note: as a Master Herbalist, I had to experience the remedies first. As a psychologist, I had to go through my own therapeutic process first. However, that may not work with all types of therapies. For instance, in homeopathic remedies "like cures like" but if you are healthy – it will cause the symptom profile to occur but you get the idea.)

"FDA officials and their colleagues want you to submit to disfiguring surgery, poisonous chemo, and burning radiation when you get cancer. But when they get cancer – well, that's different! They go to Germany to get rid of their cancer. For themselves, they prefer treatments that are more effective and don't have any side effects."

See:
http://germancancerbreakthrough.com/

"You wouldn't believe how many FDA officials or relatives or acquaintances of FDA officials come to see me as patients in Hanover. You wouldn't believe this – or directors of the American Medical Association (AMA), or American Cancer Society (ACS), or the presidents of orthodox cancer institutes. That's the fact." - Dr. Hans Nieper

See:
http://www.encognitive.com/node/1203

The warnings that come with the chemo drugs should be enough. They are incredibly toxic –

and they cause terrible problems like nausea, fatigue and hair loss. Many claim that people don't die from cancer – they die from the chemotherapy and radiation.

The reason for this is that chemotherapies are designed to address rapidly dividing cells. These cells absorb the toxic chemical which will then kill the cells. Unfortunately, cancer cells are not the only rapidly dividing cells and unlike real foods and herbs, artificial synthetic drugs do not have the capacity to differentiate between healthy cells and unhealthy cancer cells.

Among these are gastrointestinal cells (the reason for nausea, vomiting and other intestinal disturbances), parietal cells found in the stomach (which is why there is a decrease in Vitamin B12 which needs the IF transport factor released with the secretion of the stomach's hydrochloric acid), bone marrow cells (which is why people suffer a decrease in red and white blood cells), and hair follicle damage (the reason for hair loss).

In fact, the most common side effects from chemotherapy are:

- Anemia (low red blood cells)
- Fatigue

- Increased chance of bruising and bleeding

- Increased chance of infection (low white blood cells-neutrophils) – usually start in your mouth, skin, lungs, urinary tract and rectum

- Nausea and vomiting

- Hair loss

- Constipation and/or diarrhea

You'll have to agree that there is a really bizarre issue going on here. Let's take anemia for example. US TV commercials claim that Procrit is "the solution for anemia following chemotherapy". Of course, anyone with intelligence has to question any commercial but stay with me for a minute here.

First, Procrit is supposed to increase red blood cells – the ones that carry the oxygen throughout the body. This is one way of treating anemia and chronic renal failure. The more serious side effects include allergic reactions, seizures, thrombosis provoking heart attacks, strokes and pulmonary embolism. This doesn't sound too good.

Second, the usual protocol for eliminating anemia is with iron, vitamin B12, and vitamin

B9, depending on what deficiency is causing the anemia.

But let's go back to Procrit for a moment. It actually depletes all three of these substances. Further, vitamin B9 deficiency leads to an increase in homocysteine which is a marker for cardiovascular issues. How is this drug a solution?

See:
http://www.webmd.com/drugs/drug-34-Pro-crit+Inj.aspx?drugid=34&drugname=Procrit+Inj

An even worse problem is that Procrit is actually associated with "stimulated tumor growth". Wasn't this what we were struggling with in the first place?

See:
http://www.fda.gov/Drugs/DrugSafety/PostmarketDrugSafetyInformationforPatientsandProviders/ucm200297.htm

(For a list of a large range of medications and the vitamins and minerals they deplete and the subsequent side effects, go to

See:
http://choicesunlimited.ca/pharmaceuticals-

create-side-effects-and-deplete-nutrients/)

It looks like we go from cancer to anemia to hypertension (high blood pressure). So now let's look at the medications that are used for hypertension – beta blockers and calcium blockers.
Calcium blockers cause a depletion of Vitamin B12 and B9, not to mention, a shrinking brain leading to the risk of developing Alzheimer's.

See:
http://www.thefreelibrary.com/Integrating+B +vitamins+with+calcium+channel+blockers.- a0174751496

(For further information on how to recover from Alzheimer's go to:
www.choicesunlimited.ca/content/alzeheimer s-manage-it-or-eliminate-it)

Beta-blockers can cause oxygen depletion in the mitochondria and other cell functions lead- ing to loss of brain cells, depressed immune system and finally the increased risk of cancer.

Note: Other side-effects for beta blockers in- clude nausea, diarrhea, bronchospasm, dysp- nea, poor peripheral blood flow, increased Raynaud's syndrome, lowered blood pressure, heart failure, fatigue, dizziness, abnormal vi- sion, hallucinations, insomnia, nightmares, altered sugar and fat metabolism and others.

See:
http://en.wikipedia.org/wiki/Beta_blockers#
Adverse_effects

(Unfortunately, this domino effect is common throughout pharmaceutical treatments, which are why most seniors are on "cocktails" of drugs.)

But, let's get back on course here.

In addition to these commonly recognized side effects, chemotherapy also affects your body in the following ways:

- Loss of appetite

- Loss or gain of weight

- Loss of smell and taste (or everything tastes horrible)

- Destroys bone marrow so fewer blood cells are produced (red blood cells, white blood cells and platelets)

- Sore mouth, gums and throat (these can be painful and lead to even more serious problems)

- Nerve and muscle problems (neuropa-thy – a nerve issue that causes tingly, pins and needles, burning and numbing sensations especially in the hands & feet)

- Kidney and bladder irritation (both short term and long term damage)
- Intestinal and stomach problems
- Depression and anxiety
- Fatigue

See:
http://en.wikipedia.org/wiki/Chemotherapy #Adverse_effects

One of the long term effects of chemotherapy is referred to as the "chemo brain" which may be immediate but usually includes delayed onset of various cognitive dysfunctions:

- Language impairment
- Memory loss
- Poor concentration
- Poor judgment
- Poor planning capacity
- Poor reaction time

See:
http://www.urmc.rochester.edu/news/story /index.cfm?id=1963

Researchers at the University of Rochester (Medical Center) and Harvard University linked the chemotherapy 5-FU (5-fluorouracil) with cognitive degeneration. They recognized that the drugs were creating a collapse of stems cells required in the central nervous system.

"This study is the first model of a delayed degeneration syndrome that involves a global disruption of the myelin-forming cells that are essential for normal neuronal function," said Mark Noble, Ph.D. (Director of the University of Rochester Stem Cell and Regenerative Medicine Institute and senior author of the study.

See:
http://www.urmc.rochester.edu/people/?u=2 3095977

A two-year study at the James P. Wilmot Cancer Center (University of Rochester) reported that upwards of 82% of breast cancer patients reported that they suffer some form of cognitive impairment.

See:
http://www.urmc.rochester.edu/news/story /index.cfm?id=1963

Other studies have shown that between 15 and 20 % of the United States' 2.4 million female breast cancer survivors have continuing cognitive impairment years after treatment or that 50% of women had not recovered their prior level of cognitive functioning a year after treatment. (Dr. Tanton, Taking the Mystery Out of Cancer, p.28)

Other researchers have recognized more specific neural mechanisms. For instance, Noble's work explored the impact of chemotherapy on the neural myelination (insulation on the stem of the neurons that allows the neuron to release neurotransmitter). This important insulation, like the rest of the body, is being constantly renewed. The brain requires a specific type of cell to regenerate the myelination called oligodendrocytes.

Dr. Noble's team found that three common chemotherapy drugs damaged these oligodendrocytes and the stem cells from which emerged, so greatly that they had all but disappeared even six months after the therapy.

(Retrieved from http://www.sciencedaily.com/releases/2008/04/080422103947.htm).

In some cases, neural dysfunction may extend to:
1. Seizures
2. Vision loss
3. Dementia

Children

When it comes to the effect of cancer treatment on children the research is even more depressing.

The following was a study at Emory University. What they reported was that repeated studies revealed that children who have received radiation, chemotherapy and other such treatments lived shorter lives and developed severe conditions.

"As a result of their curative therapies, childhood cancer survivors face an increased risk of morbidity and mortality," the researchers wrote. Nearly 75 percent of such children develop a chronic health condition within 30 years of diagnosis, while 42.4 percent develop severe, disabling or life threatening health conditions.

See:
http://www.diabetes-and-diabetic-dit.com/article/radiation_increase_diabetes_risk.htm
http://www.ncbi.nlm.nih.gov/pubmed/20056636

References:
http://www.naturalnews.com/z028032_radiation_therapy_diabetes.html:

See:
http://www.medicinenet.com/epoetin_alfa/article.htm

http://www.onlineholistichealth.com/vitamin-b12-deficiency/
http://www.rxlist.com/procrit-drug/patient-images-side-effects.htm#sideeffects

Baselt, R. Disposition of Toxic Drugs and Chemicals in Man, 8th edition, Biomedical Publications, Foster City, CA, 2008, pp. 547-549.

Edwards, Jim (August 17, 2009), Drug Rep in $3B Procrit Case: "80% of My Sales Were Medicare Fraud"; Carried $400K in "Cash",

(CBS news,
http://www.cbsnews.com/8301-505123_162-42842558/drug-rep-in-3b-procrit-case-80-of-my-sales-were-medicare-fraud-carried-400k-in-cash/)

Engelberg, Alfred B. et al., Balancing innovation, access, and profits -- marketing exclusivity for biologics, N Engl J Med 361:1917
Hardell L, Walker MJ, Walhjalt B, Friedman LS, Richter ED (March 2007). "Secret ties to industry and conflicting interests in cancer research". Am. J. Ind. Med. 50 (3): 227–33.
Napoli, Maryann (October 5, 2011), Whistle-

blower's story: New book reviewed

Center for Medical Consumers,
http://medicalconsumers.org/2011/10/05/w
histleblowers-story-new-book-reviewed/

Walsh, G, Spada, S. "Epogen/Procrit" in: Direc-
tory of approved biopharmaceutical products.
CRC Press, 2005, pp.39-41.

SEVEN

What do some of the specialists say?

Now let's look at what a few of the specialists say. Let me remind you, however, that these individuals listed below are only a few of a huge and growing number of specialists who are turning to functional health in their practices and learning how to work with the body rather than against it. Consider the following quotes from medical professionals.

Dr. Mark Roth:
"The reason breast cancer and other malignancies often return aggressively after treatment is that when tumor cells die under assault from chemotherapy and radiation, they give off substances that can reactivate a special set of master cells known as cancer stem cells," Dr. Wicha said in an interview.

Dr. Wicha's lab has found that inflammatory molecules secreted by dying tumor cells can hook up with the stem cells and cause them, in effect, to come out of hibernation. Adult stem cells exist in most tissues, and go into action to repair damage from wounds or infections. In cancer, they can mutate and no longer obey normal bodily signals to stop growing, Dr. Wicha said.

He and other researchers say that even when chemotherapy and radiation cause tumors to shrink dramatically, these stem cells can stay alive, living "under the radar" until they are once again spurred into action. They also believe stem cells are probably the ones that break away from an original tumor and cause cancer to spread elsewhere in the body.

See:
http://www.postgazette.com/pg/10055/1038 056-114.stm

In Suzanne Somers book, Knockout, she quotes Dr. Nicholas Gonzalez, M.D., saying, "The fact of the matter is that for all the major cancer killers – metastatic breast, lung, prostate, and pancreatic – chemotherapy does absolutely nothing... zero". (Suzanne Somers, Knockout, 2009, p. 95)

Dr. Mercola has reported numerous interviews with people in the "cancer industry" and claims that, "Most conventional cancer treatments tend to add insult to injury by doing more harm than good – a fact that has been largely swept under the rug by the medical industry.

The real culprits – the underlying causes – are completely ignored, and that is, I believe, the root of the problem. The cancer industry has become a massive for-profit business that is doing everything in its power to maintain the status quo. It is, quite simply, not interested in truly reducing cancer rates; it's interested in treating cancer. From that perspective, the more cancer cases the better... Even many on-cologists, whom most regard as the go-to spe-cialist upon receiving a cancer diagnosis, may be better described as chemotherapy specialists than cancer specialists."

May Alleviate Cancer Without Chemo, But it's Forbidden, June 10 2012-

See:
http://articles.mercola.com/sites/articles/arc hive/2012/06/10/dr-mercola-on-ric-schiff.aspx

"Most cancer patients in this country die of chemotherapy. Chemotherapy does not elimi-nate breast, colon, or lung cancers. This fact has been documented for over a decade. Yet doc-tors still use chemotherapy for these tumors. Women with breast cancer are likely to die faster with chemo than without it." Dr. Allan Levin.

See:
http://www.cancerarchy.com/nucleus/index.
php?catid=8

A recent January edition of the New York Times published a startling and ground breaking series of reports by investigative reporter Walt Bogdanich, who has uncovered case after case of people who suffered devastating consequences – including horrendously painful, torture-like deaths – because of medical mistakes related to radiation treatment. In response to these articles, the American Association of Physicists in Medicine (AAPM) just issued a statement saying the group and its members "deeply regret that these events have occurred, and we continue to work hard to reduce the likelihood of similar events in the future." S.L. Baker

See:
http://www.naturalnews.com/z028127_radiat
ion_therapy_medical_mistakes.html

Dr. Tanton states: "The theory that it's perfectly okay to destroy your body (and brain), in an attempt to somehow kill the cancer, is based solely on deception. We need to take more responsibility for our own health. If the advice you receive doesn't seem logical, such as exposing your body to the highly toxic radiation and chemotherapy "capable of causing cancer", question the wisdom considering such a dangerous therapy – even if it were free! As you are likely aware, it's far from free. In fact it's the most expensive therapy, as well as the most toxic therapy, for a disease that can be easily be prevented." (Dr. Tanton, Taking The Mystery Out of Cancer, 2011, p. 39)

"The success rate of most chemotherapy is appalling. There is no scientific evidence for its ability to extend in any appreciable way the lives of patients suffering from the most common organic cancers. Chemotherapy for malignancies too advanced for surgery, which accounts for 80% of all cancers, is a scientific wasteland."
Dr. Ulrich Abel, 1990

See:
http://www.cancerarchy.com/nucleus/index.php?catid=8

The New England Journal of Medicine Reports, "The War on Cancer Is a Failure: Despite $30 billion spent on research and treatments since 1970, cancer remains "undefeated" with a death rate not lower but 6% higher in 1997 than 1970." -John C. Bailar III, M.D., Ph.D., and Heather L. Gornik, M.H.S., Department of Health Studies, University of Chicago, Illinois. "The war against cancer is far from over," states Dr. Bailar. "The effect of new treatments for cancer on mortality has been largely disappointing."

See:
http://www.cancerarchy.com/nucleus/index.php?catid=8

"..chemotherapy's success record is dismal. It can achieve remissions in about 7% of all human cancers; for an additional 15% of cases, survival can be "prolonged" beyond the point at which death would be expected without treatment. This type of survival is not the same as a cure or even restored quality of life." -John Diamond, M.D.

See:
http://www.cancerarchy.com/nucleus/index.php?catid=8

"I wouldn't have chemotherapy and radiation because I'm not interested in therapies that cripple the immune system, and, in my opinion, virtually ensure failure for the majority of cancer patients." -Dr. Julian Whitaker, M.D.

See:
http://www.cancerarchy.com/nucleus/index.php?catid=8

Dr. Frank Shallenberger says, "Doctors are finally realizing that most people have cancer in their body. But it's latent – or hidden – cancer." Then he goes on to explain, "The existence of latent cancers is very reassuring. They clearly demonstrate how effective a healthy immune system can be in stopping cancer. It's so effective that the great majority of latent cancers never go on to become full-blown cancers. And that's good news." (Dr. Frank Shallenberger's Real Cures newsletter, March 2011, vol. 10, No. 3).

"Finding a cure for cancer is absolutely contra-indicated by the profits of the cancer industry's chemotherapy, radiation, and surgery cash trough." -Dr. Diamond, M.D.

See:
http://www.cancerarchy.com/nucleus/index.php?catid=8

"We have a multi-billion dollar industry that is killing people, right and left, for financial gain. Their idea of research is to see whether two doses of this poison is better than three doses of that poison." – Dr. Glen Warner, M.D., on-cologist.

See:
http://www.cancerarchy.com/nucleus/index.php?catid=8

"If you can shrink the tumor 50% or more for

28 days you have got the FDA's definition of an active drug. That is called a response rate, so you have a response...(but) when you look to see if there is any life prolongation from taking this treatment, what you find is all kinds of hocus pocus and song and dance about the disease-free survival, and this and that. In the end there is no proof that chemotherapy in the vast majority of cases actually extends life, and this is the GREAT LIE about chemotherapy, that somehow there is a correlation between shrinking a tumor and extending the life of the patient." -Ralph Moss

See:
http://www.cancerarchy.com/nucleus/index.php?catid=8

Even people working with the drugs are being exposed to highly toxic environments that put them at risk. Special gowns, double layer gloves, special ventilation hoods, respirators and face shields have been recommended when administering these toxic treatments. (2004, National Institute for Occupational Safety and Health, NIOSH, US). In Dr. Tanton's book, Taking the Mystery Out of Cancer, 2011, he records what Dr. Thomas (NIOSH biologist) said about finding the chemotherapy drugs in the blood and urine of the nurses and other health care workers:

"Most workplace surfaces are contaminated with the drugs being prepared and used in that area. Bodily fluids from patients receiving these drugs contain levels of chemotherapy agents that are even more biologically active than the original drugs. While it's thought that skin exposure is currently the primary route of exposure for health care workers, it's possible they could be exposed from working with chemotherapy patients as well." (Dr. Tanton. Taking the Mystery out of Cancer. 2011, p. 31)

The challenge for alternative practitioners is that it is usually when the conventional methods have failed that cancer patients go to an alternative physician. Yet by this time the situation has digressed enormously, the cancer has metastasized and the drugs have done so much damage that the alternative physician has little to work with.

However, if the patient had come to the alternative practitioner in the beginning the results would have been excellent. Are physicians aware of these options? Are they taught that alternative procedures are unscientific? How much money do the physicians make providing these therapies that are so toxic with such poor results? In the US, oncologists' incomes come from the commissions on chemo drugs and the reimbursement for surgery.

In Canada, I am told by many accountants, that what physicians get paid from pharmaceutical companies far outweighs what they get paid through the government medical program.

The Life Extension Foundation built a large facility to treat cancer patients with non-toxic therapies but every oncologist that they approached wanted to know what the commissions were that they would make on the chemo drugs. No chemo drugs, no commission, so no one came. They have a beautiful site with a lot of information:

See:
http://www.lef.org/protocols/cancer/cancer_adjuvant_therapy_01.htm

Interesting research came out last year. The statistics given to insurance companies reflected that for the first time there was an increase in the recovery rates for cancer sufferers. What they failed to mention was that there was a significant and corresponding increase in the number of cancer patients who chose to have treatments through alternative medicine.

EIGHT

Ways to make medications worse

Non-nutritious food
If the body requires nutrients to make:

- Cells
- Neurons
- Skin
- Organs
- Muscles
- Bones
- Proteins
- Enzymes
- Hormones
- Neurotransmitters
- And more...

Then it only makes sense we need to have good healthy food.

However, much of our "food" in North America is:

1. Man-made
2. Over-processed
3. Micro-waved
4. GMO (genetically modified organism)

And loaded with:

- Sweeteners (HFCS, Aspartame, Nu-traSweet, etc.)
- Preservatives
- Colorings
- High fructose corn syrup
- Artificial and natural flavorings (natural flavorings are loaded with artificial chemicals as well).

And even if it is real food, it is loaded with:

- Pesticides
- Herbicides
- Vaccinations
- Growth hormones

And even if it is called organic, real food, we have to look at whether there were enough real nutrients in the soil so that we get the nutrients we need out of the food.

For instance, if we take a serving of broccoli from fifty years ago and profile the nutrients, we would have to consume twenty-two servings today to make up the same nutrient profile! Food simply isn't what it used to be.

Now our bodies require even more nutrients because we have to work with the much higher level of toxicities in our bodies and in our daily environments.

And then there are the artificial sweeteners...

NutraSweet, a.k.a. Aspartame, is a great example to start with. NutraSweet is an artificial sweetener that has evoked a lot of controversy. Many claims indicate that it turns into formaldehyde (the embalming fluid is that is put on dead bodies – paralyzing any activity – in order to preserve them for autopsy) in the body. It is known for increasing the risk of brain cancers and interacting with medications and vaccinations in such a manner that it increases their already established risk factor.

See:
http://en.wikipedia.org/wiki/Aspartame

http://www.caloriecontrol.org/articles-and-video/feature-articles/internet-myths-about-aspartame

http://www.bio.net/bionet/mm/neur-sci/1999-January/036300.html

The following is a sampling of issues identified on various websites and books:

Taken from *Aspartame - Is It Safe? by H J Roberts MD, page 226* **Dr.** Roberts discusses Dr Lampert's findings regarding brain tumor studies. He was surprised at the how large the tumors were in the NutraSweet-fed rats.

Or the article wherein the FDA reviewed the data from a 2 year study on male and female Sprague-Dawley rats fed various amounts of aspartame. (G. D. Searle and Co., 1973b). The FDA inquiry board concluded that aspartame was a possible carcinogen: "The incidence of brain neoplasms in aspartame-fed rats was greater than that in controls, ..." *Diet Nutrition Cancer by National Research Council, page311*

See:
http://www.nap.edu/catalog.php?record_id=371

There are several hypotheses that have been presented to account for cancer in animals fed aspartame. Several possibilities explain the high rate of cancer in these animals.

For instance, the body metabolizes aspartame into a substance called diketopiperizine or DKP. The chemical structure of DKP resembles a whole group of cancer causing chemicals.

Or the fact that Aspartame contains methanol, which is known to break down in the body into formaldehyde and formic acid. Studies have shown that formaldehyde tends to accumulate near DNA, causing serious accumulative damage.

So while you may not drink a lot of soda on a given day, even drinking one diet soda a day can cause formaldehyde buildup in cells, so that the amount of the toxin increases daily. *Health And Nutrition Secrets by Russell L Blaylock MD, page 197*

...and aspartame (NutraSweet) .... Some experts suspect them of promoting cancer and having toxic effects on the nervous system. You are much better off eating moderate amounts of sugar than any of these unnatural compounds. *8 Weeks To Optimum Health By Andrew Weil MD, page 51*

Dr Roberts recognizes and explores the possibility of whether brain tumors are really on the rise or are they just better diagnosed today. He claims that with the rise in AIDS and the corresponding immune depression – one would expect to see an increase. His conclusion is that there is also a dramatic rise in individuals without AIDS, and rather than immune disorders accounting for the increase...he believes it is the significant increase in the use of Aspartame. *Excitotoxins by Russell L Blaylock MD, page 215 Aspartame and other disorders*

NINE

Cancer and Surgery

Surgery is often the recommended course of action when dealing with cancerous tumors. However, reports of surgical removal of tumors is very misleading because even when the medical experts claim they were successful and "got all the tumor", they have no idea whether they got all of the cancer. Claims of this kind are deceptive.

Cancer tumors tend to grow in spurts and then rest in a maintenance stage for prolonged periods. During this prolonged stage, pieces of the tumor break apart and move into the blood and lymph system and flow throughout the body. This is why, even if the tumor was entirely removed, it does not mean that all the cancer was removed.

British Journal of Surgery claimed that, "surgical operations are not always beneficial to patients...a year after their surgeries, 17 percent of patients reported more pain than before, 14 percent indicated reduced functional ability and 16 percent said their mental states had declined."

See:
http://www.bjs.co.uk/view/0/podcasts.html

A study reported in the Journal of the American Medical Association (JAMA) found that, "Two to 3 years after breast cancer treatment, persistent pain and sensory disturbances remain clinically significant problems ...persistent post-surgical pain has been demonstrated to be clinically relevant in 10% to 50% of patients undergoing various common operations..." Mastectomies, breast conserving surgeries, radiation treatments, chemotherapy, and lymph node dissection were among the treatments women in the study had received.

See:
(http://jama.jamanetwork.com/article.aspx?ar ticleid=184861)

Peripheral drugs can also be a big problem. For instance, the anesthesia used for surgery is not only toxic to the brain but suppress the immune system – the system you need to be highly functioning to protect you not only from the cancer but from possible infections due to the surgical process itself. So normally we want the NK (Natural Killer cells) to be up and functioning at their utmost best but now they are suppressed which allows the cancer cells to go undetected.

Here is another little-known fact. The types of molecules we produce after surgery to help the wound to heal actually help cancer cells. First, the adhesion molecules which help the wound to close also help the cancer cells adhere to the blood walls and to each other, thus making another tumor. Apparently, after surgery, the increase of cancer cells binding to the blood vessel walls is about 250%. This is not something you want.

In addition, after surgery we also produce more VEGF (vascular endothelium growth factor). This allows for the creation (angiogenesis) of new capillaries to support the new cell growth but this same VEGF is utilized by the cancer cells to promote themselves.

The morphine, a commonly used pain-killer after surgery, can actually promote cancer as well. Dr. Howenstine claims that, "many cancers have morphine receptors that speed up the growth of cancer when morphine or its derivatives are used to treat pain".

See:
www.newswithviews.com/Howenstine/james62.htm

The other challenge with surgery is the need for a blood transfusion. Dr. David Williams claims that current research reveals that the odds of having any kind of infection is 3x greater in any patient who receives a blood transfusion compared to a patient to who didn't. Further, he wrote that patients who received blood transfusions were five times more likely to die within 100 days of their operation compared to those who did not. (Am Heart Journal 06; 252(6): 1028-1034).

This is presumably due to the fact that our blood not only contains hundreds of antigens (they trigger an immune response) and tumor antigens but also pathogens, allergens, toxicities, pollutants and auto antigens (causing auto immune disease). So the transfusion may not only end up imposing an excessive task on the already compromised immune system but also may leave us with an autoimmune disease. (Dr. David G. Williams' Unabridged Library of Medical Lies, 2009, pp. 44-45)

As a herbalist, I know that there are various ways of helping the healing take place so that a transfusion is not required. For instance, cayenne pepper and horse chestnut can be used. Cayenne pepper not only improves peripheral blood circulation but also has the intelligence to rapidly eliminate unwanted blood loss during surgery while horse chestnut is an astringent that is utilized to do the repair work. The reason these simple, cheap effective methods are not used? They are natural and cannot be patented – therefore there is no money to be made by drug corporations.

Another practice that benefits the cancer more than you – is by doing an autopsy. You do an autopsy to see if the tumor is actually carcinogenic – but in doing so you have broken the protein coating that encloses the cancer and now you have increased the tumor's ability to metastasize.

Due to the fact that surgery can actually be of such benefit to the cancer, many alternative practitioners will suggest that if you need surgery you should actually wait until after the cancer has been killed and after you have allowed time for the immune system to rebuild. Of course, by this time you won't likely need the surgery.

As many have noted, there used to be a requirement that physicians take the Hippocratic oath, which says, First Do No Harm. Unfortunately, between the grip of pharmaceutical control and the changes to the medical profession, this oath has somehow become lost.

TEN

Cancer and Statistics

Statistics on cancer can be very depressing.

Take for instance the fact that tens of millions of dollars have been committed to fighting cancer yet the success rate is only 2.1%. (Note that reads two point one percent NOT twenty-one percent.)

Where does all that money go? All that money raised by well-meaning charitable organizations and interest groups ends up somewhere, but where? For one thing, the American Cancer Association is the richest association in the world yet people are still walking and running and doing whatever they can to raise funds for more cancer research!

In addition, this association is known to buy off people who do successful research and/or simply ignore other protocols that have been proven to work. Why? Well, usually because the pharmaceutical companies can't make money utilizing natural foods and herbs. It's all about the money to be made.

See:
http://www.preventcancer.com/losing/acs/
wealthiest_links.htm

Twenty thousand people die of cancer daily.
This translates into eight million deaths annu-
ally.

See:
http://www.allnurses.com/nursing-news/20-
000-people-268319.html

At the beginning of the last century one in
twenty people was diagnosed with cancer. By
1940 the statistic had moved to one in sixteen
people. Today the statistics show that one person in three is now diagnosed with this disease.

As so many people have asked, where has all
the money gone?

That's a good question.

ELEVEN

Cancer and Money

There are many who have had the courage to stand up and speak out about what the FDA and other organizations are actually doing, what they fail to do and who pays the wages. These organizations do not appear to be protecting the general public's physiological or psychological health but rather, protecting the wealth of a very few.

"The FDA is the chief agency in charge of protecting and promoting Americans' health and safety." But in 10 stunning, true stories in his book, The Politics of Healing, former New York State assemblyman, Daniel Haley describes how the FDA has suppressed and banned natural health cures – eight of them for cancer.

The FDA even admitted that one of these treatments, discovered by Dr. Stanislaw Burzynski, was successful with some of the most incurable forms of cancer. How many people have died while the FDA denied them cancer treatments that work?

See:
http://articles.mercola.com/sites/articles/arc hive/2011/08/06/why-we-dont-have-a-cure-for-cancer-yet-or-do-we.aspx

The following is a very short list of the various health practitioners and others who are willing to challenge the FDA and other associations that claim they are protecting our health:

Dr. WC Douglass   www.healthiertalk.com

Dr. Mark Hyman   www.drhyman.com

Dr. Mercola   www.mercola.com

Dr. Al Sears   www.healthiertalk.com

Dr. David Tanton   www.drtanto.com

Dr. Julian Whitaker   www.youtube.com/-watch?v=kxLSUaKb4pI

Jenny Thompson   www.hsionline.com

Jon Christian Ryter

http://www.jonchristianryter.com/

Kevin Trudeau

www.ktradionetwork.com (very controversial)

http://www.forhealthfreedom.org/Publicatio ns/Monopoly/wsj-970602.html

www.cancerinform.org/kids1.html

www.naturalnews.com

But let's take a look at some of these issues and treatments now ourselves.

Avastin, a.k.a. Bevacizumab, is a chemotherapy that is considered a bestseller. It will cost the patient about $8000 per month if he is paying for it and it is prescribed even though it has not been proven to extend life or even improve the quality of life.

However, the shares in the company increased 25% when it was announced that Avastin showed promise in keeping lung cancer patients alive. Note that nothing about the quality of life was mentioned. According to Mercola, the drug was noted as potentially fatal, causing slow wound healing, stroke, hypertension, gastro-intestinal perforation hemorrhage, severe kidney malfunction, and more.

http://articles.mercola.com/sites/articles/archive/2010/08/23/why-does-medicinehave-to-profit-so-much-and-kill-cancer-victims-prematurely.aspx

As many have already questioned, how long are people and corporations and countries going to stand by and allow big pharmaceutical companies to deplete our health and our wealth?

With an almost universal economic crisis

occurring, can we afford to allow "Big Pharma" to continue to deplete our resources? Our health? Our wealth? Can the government continue to allow this to function? It is shocking to realize that apparently over 50% of the U.S. Government, the Senate represents pharmaceutical companies.

http://endthelie.com/2012/04/18/18-venn-diagrams-showing-how-corrupted-american-democracy-really-is/#axzz2F2IuASrl

What about the Cancer Societies? People across North America are willing to walk, run, paddle and buy the pink ribbon on anything to support cancer research but where does the money actually go?

According to an article printed by Dr. Epstein, MD, in 1988 the American Cancer Society (ACS), here is an indication. Let's look at some of the cross overs between government and pharmaceutical companies...

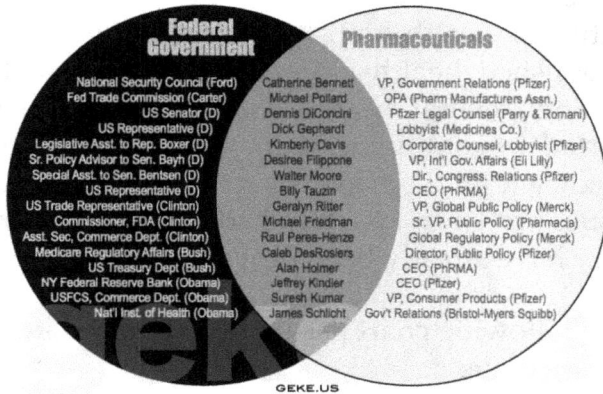

Federal Government

National Security Council (Ford)
Fed Trade Commission (Carter)
US Senator (D)
US Representative (D)
Legislative Asst. to Rep. Boxer (D)
Sr. Policy Advisor to Sen. Bayh (D)
Special Asst. to Sen. Bentsen (D)
US Representative (D)
US Trade Representative (Clinton)
Commissioner, FDA (Clinton)
Asst. Sec, Commerce Dept. (Clinton)
Medicare Regulatory Affairs (Bush)
US Treasury Dept (Bush)
NY Federal Reserve Bank (Obama)
USFCS, Commerce Dept. (Obama)
Nat'l Inst. of Health (Obama)

Catherine Bennett
Michael Pollard
Dennis DiConcini
Dick Gephardt
Kimberly Davis
Desiree Filippone
Walter Moore
Billy Tauzin
Geralyn Ritter
Michael Friedman
Raul Perea-Henze
Caleb DesRosiers
Alan Holmer
Jeffrey Kindler
Suresh Kumar
James Schlicht

Pharmaceuticals

VP, Government Relations (Pfizer)
OPA (Pharm Manufacturers Assn.)
Pfizer Legal Counsel (Parry & Romani)
Lobbyist (Medicines Co.)
Corporate Counsel, Lobbyist (Pfizer)
VP, Int'l Gov. Affairs (Eli Lilly)
Dir., Congress. Relations (Pfizer)
CEO (PhRMA)
VP, Global Public Policy (Merck)
Sr. VP, Public Policy (Pharmacia)
Global Regulatory Policy (Merck)
Director, Public Policy (Pfizer)
CEO (PhRMA)
CEO (Pfizer)
VP, Consumer Products (Pfizer)
Gov't Relations (Bristol-Myers Squibb)

GEKE.US

This is used with permission from:
http://endthelie.com/2012/04/18/18-venn-diagrams-showing-how-corrupted-american-democracy-really-is/#axzz1zVGJNDpe

This site has a series of eighteen Venn diagrams showing how corrupted American "democracy" really is.

See:
http://EndtheLie.com/2012/04/18/18-venn-diagrams-showing-how-corrupted-american-democracy-really-is/#ixzz1zVHv8hcg

Further, these same officials also stand on the executive boards of the other companies depleting our health such as Monsanto, the chief company producing the GMOs, Genetically Modified Organisms. While knowing that these engineered "foods" would create havoc with our health both by exacerbating already established health issues like cancer and depleting general health, they have been supported in continuing their work. GMOs were predicted by the scientists to create new health issues we hadn't to date had to deal with and they have already been proven right.

The following chart has been on several sites: Dr. Mercola:
http://www.abovetopsecret.com/forum/thread778572/pg1

http://media.mercola.com/ImageServer/public/2012/january/study1-big.jpg

http://www.sallyhomemaker.com/journal/corrupt-the-governments-revolving-door-with-monsanto/

http://www.abovetopsecret.com/forum/thread778572/pg1

Monsanto Position	Individual	Federal Government Position
Head of Government Affairs for Genetech, (Now Monsanto)	David Beier	Chief Domestic Policy Advisor to Vice President Gore
Worked for Monsanto's	William Conlon	Department of Justice

Legal Team Worked for Monsanto's Legal Team	Sam Skinner	Department of Justice
Executive Vice President and Chief Technology Officer	Robert Fraley	Serves as advisor in public agencies, including the USDA, among others
Senior Vice President for Clinical Affairs at G.D. Searle & Co (Merged with Monsanto)	Michael A. Friedman	Acting Commissioner of the FDA
Director of International Government Affairs	Marcia Hale	Asst. to Pres. Clinton and Director of Governmental Affairs
Consultant to Searle's (Merged with Monsanto) Public Relations Firm	Arthur Hull Hayes	Previously was FDA Commissioner
Director of ESH Quality & Compliance	John L. Henshaw	Senior Advisor to U.S. Secretary of Labor
Vice President of Product and Technology Cooperation	Rob Horsch	Advisor to the National Science Foundation and the Dept. of Energy
Board of Direc-	Michael	U.S. Secretary of

tors, also represented Monsanto as a lawyer	Kantor	Commerce
Monsanto Board Member	Gwendolyn S. King	Commissioner of SSA 1989-1992
CEO of Monsanto for 14 years	Richard J. Mahoney	Served as Director of U.S. Soviet, Japanese and Korean Trade Councils, a Member of the U.S. Government Trade Policy Committee
Oversaw the Approval of rBGH, was a top Monsanto scientist	Margaret Miller	In 1991, Margaret was appointed Deputy Director of the FDA
Sits on Monsanto's Board of Directors, previously a Monsanto Animal Specialist	George Poste	In 2002, Poste was appointed head of Bioterrorism division of Homeland Security
Member of the Monsanto Board of Directors	William D. Ruckelshaus	In 1970, he was the first Chief Administrator for the EPA, later the acting director of the FBI, then Deputy U.S. Attorney General
Previous CEO	Donald	Appointed to

of Searle (Merged with Monsanto), he successfully had aspartame legalized while in that position.	Rumsfeld	Secretary of Defense in 1975, then appointed to the same position again in 2000
Worked on Monsanto-funded rBGH in connection with her graduate work at Cornell University	Suzanne Sechen	FDA Reviewer on Scientific Data
Previously the President and COO of Monsanto, Chairman and CEO of Nutrasweet, and Chairman and CEO of Monsanto	Robert B. Shapiro	Previously served on President's Advisory Committee on Trade Policy and on the White House Domestic Policy Review of Industrial Innovation
Former Vice President of CropLife America, which represented Monsanto	Islam Siddiqui	Chief Agricultural Negotiator for the Office of the U.S. Trade Representative
Former Attorney for Monsanto for seven years, previous	Michael Taylor	Former FDA Deputy Commission for Policy. In 2010, appoint-

head of the Monsanto Washington, D.C. office		ed by the FDA as a senior advisor to the FDA Commissioner.
Previous Monsanto Researcher in charge of the Manhattan Project, creating the atomic bomb. Later became Monsanto's Chairman of the Board.	Dr. Charles Thomas	Previously served as a consultant to the National Security Council and as a U.S. Representative to the United Nations' Atomic Energy Commission
Former lawyer for Monsanto, a notorious chemical polluter.	Clarence Thomas	In 1991, was appointed to the U.S. Supreme Court
Previously served on the Board of Directors of Calgene, a Monsanto Biotech subsidiary.	Anne Veneman	In 2001, was appointed head of the USDA
Former Staff Lawyer with Monsanto in Washington, D.C.	Jack Watson	Chief of Staff to Pres. Jimmy Carter
Hired by Mon-	Seth Wax-	Former U.S. So-

The company that accounts for nearly half of the chemotherapy sales in the world – Bristol-Meyers Squibb.

Chairman of the board of Bristol-Meyers Squibb - Richard L. Gelb.

Mr. Gelb's other job? Vice Chairman, Board of Overseers, Board of Managers, and Memorial Sloan-Kettering Cancer Center.

Former Chairman, Memorial Sloan-Kettering's Board of Overseers, Board of Managers - John S. Reed.

Reed's other job? Director, Philip Morris (the tobacco company).

Director, Ivax, Inc. (Chemotherapy company) – Samuel Broder.

Broder's other job (until 1995)? Executive Director, National Cancer Institute.

See:
http://www.cancerarchy.com/nucleus/index.php?catid=8

It doesn't take much imagination to conclude that there is something wrong with this picture.

TWELVE

Cancer and Legalities and your rights

Different countries have different legal issues that they may have to contend with when dealing with medical services. Even within a country, there may be differences from province to province or state to state.

What we need to look at is what happens when an oncologist is really a chemotherapy specialist not a cancer specialist.

When it is questionable whether they understand what the chemotherapy is doing to the cancer cells, the healthy cells, the glial cells, the liver, and more; when it is possible for a judge to decide who you or your child has to go to, to get your treatment; when it is well known that no strides in healing cancer have been made but massive strides in making money have; when there are well-documented cures that have been shelved, ignored or eliminated through judicial mandates, what is a patient to do?

One has to question system that operates in this way.

When it is reported that the judges of the FDA are actually paid for by the pharmaceutical companies and that more than half of the U.S. senators represent pharmaceutical companies and not the people, something is wrong.

When it is reported that oncologists' paychecks are made up of 80% commission on toxic chemotherapies that are not helping people, one has to question the system.

Campbell, Colin. The China Study. 2004
Trudeau, Kevin. Natural Cures. 2005.
Tanton, David. Taking the Mystery Out of Cancer. 2011

See:
www.mercola.com
www.natural news.com
www.drlwilson.com

Consider the following cases:

Daniel Hauser is a teen whose mother tried to take him out of the country to get alternative rather than conventional chemotherapy. She was threatened with jail when the judge claimed that she had to abide by the oncologist's directives.

Abraham Cherrix, a 16 year-old teen who refused a second round of chemo, claiming that

the first round had almost killed him. Manda-
tory chemotherapy was dropped from the
prosecutor's case.

Both of these boys are healthy today. The difference lies in the process. Abraham got to
work with a holistic physician who addressed
his whole body-mind continuum and never
had to suffer the toxic chemo that almost destroyed his immune system.

See:

http://www.newcancerstrategy.com/blog/th
e-courts-vs-medical-freedom-a-look-back-at-
cherrix-and-hauser.html

When Healing Becomes a Crime, was written
in 2000, by Kenny Ausubel. In the book, he
identifies that incompetent people or children
don't have rights. We, the people, are considered to be incompetent because we did not
study a curriculum designed by pharmaceutical companies; we do not follow a procedure
and protocol book designed by pharmaceutical
companies. We do not get paid directly or indirectly by the pharmaceutical companies.

Whereas, the medical community is considered
to be competent and has rights because they
followed a curriculum that the pharmaceutical
companies designed and work in accordance
with a protocol and procedure manual that the

pharmaceutical companies designed. When they are trained on "evidence-based medicine" that frequently is simply hypothesis lacking evidence; when the medical community is controlled by the pharmaceutical companies and money; when they have no training in food, nutrients, herbs and basic molecular, functional biology – who is really competent enough to make these kinds of decisions?

In her book, Suzanne Somers acknowledged that six physicians claimed that she had serious cancer throughout her body and required chemotherapy immediately, based on an MRI scan. All six oncologists were wrong! They did some research; found some alternative options; and then wrote the book: Knockout: Interviews with Doctors Who Are Curing Cancer and How to Prevent It in the First Place.

I have talked with senior doctors who read such scans and interpret them and they all say it is a very difficult art that has no absolutes. Further, the research on the accuracy of the various tools in diagnosing varies widely, between MRI, MRI with or without DWI, PET, CT, PET/CT. The accuracies seem to range from 56% to 92%. That is sure one heck of a range when dealing with cancer tumors.

Thankfully, more and more physicians are becoming functional physicians, which simply

mean they are moving away from the pharmaceuticals and into nutrition and herbs and supplements as they begin to understand the basic
nutrients the body requires in order to function.

See:

http://www.surgisphere.com/SurgRad/issue
s/volume-2/1-april-2011-pages-111-206/170-
original-article-petct-whole-body-mri-and-
whole-body-ct-in-the-diagnosis-staging-and-
follow-up-of-malignancy.html

http://www.ncbi.nlm.nih.gov/pmc/articles/
PMC2023947/

THIRTEEN

How cancer cells operate

There are a number of considerations that make cancer cells different from other cells.

1) Apoptosis is turned off at a genetic level.

> What does this mean? The rest of the cells in your body have a "pre-programmed cell death" called apoptosis. This mechanism is turned off in cancer cells so the cells keep dividing but never dying.

> a) Solution: We need to turn apoptosis back on and we now know we can do this with foods and herbs.

2) Cancer cell membranes have a different "potentiation".

> This means they take in glucose and not oxygen. Cancer cells are anaerobic and do not like oxygen.

> a) Solution: We need to change the membrane potentiation of cancer cells and

we now know we can do this with foods and herbs.

3) Because of the high levels of glucose, amongst other issues, cancer cells are very acidic.

This allows them to function well with the typical acidic forming diet in North America.

a) Solution: We need to take in an alkalizing diet of food, water, minerals and herbs.

b) We need to eliminate the acidic foods in our bodies. For instance, the sugars, the sodas, coffee, medications, alcohol, acidic water (tap water legally has to have a pH of 5; bottled water can have a pH as low as 2.2!).

4) These anaerobic cancer cells produce energy utilizing the fermentation, lactic acid process.

The resulting low pH or acidic environment also contributes to the depletion of oxygen. (This process also causes pain. When we stretch and utilize muscles for the first time, for instance, the first time you go skiing in the winter, or the first time you work in the garden in the spring, you tend to feel achy and sore the next day. This is because the muscles lacked sufficient oxygen and started to engage in the lactic acid cycle instead. The result is pain. It is this lactic acid that cancer cells produce.

a) Solutions: we need to flush the system with oxygen and we can do this with supplements and alkaline water and food.

   i) Super Phytoplankton is a good source for this. See Chapter 14 for more.

   ii) Rhodiola is also a good herb to increase both oxygen diffusion and increase the efficiency of oxygen utilization. In addition, it has the added benefit of being a good anti-oxidant.

   http://www.raysahelian.com/rhodiola.html

Would you believe chemotherapy also depletes red blood cells and oxygen?

See:
http://www.lymphomainfo.net/tests/bloodcounts.html

1) We are all familiar with dehydration but it is important to realize that while everything may appear normal, the smallest of the arteries, called capillaries, may be damaged due to dehydration and these are the vessels to provide nutrient and oxygen to the cells.

   a) Solutions: Do not drink during a meal or you will dilute the necessary enzymes required to digest a meal.

   b) Drink prior to a meal to help recognize when you are full but to get the necessary oxygen throughout the body.

2) Natural hormones, when in excess, can also cause oxygen depletion. For instance, if there is an excess of estrogens in the body these will cause the heart to stiffen.

   a) Solution: One molecule we know that regulates estrogens in the body is glutathione. Increase the glutathione and the liver will regulate the necessary levels of estrogen.

3) We also have to be aware of the medications that also deplete oxygen in the body, like blood pressure medications, anticoagulants and diuretic medication.

a) Solution: Go to http://choicesunlimited.ca/pharm aceuticals-create-side-effects-and-deplete-nutrients/ to find a list of medications and the nutrients that each depletes. You have the choices of either utilizing something different or compensating for the nutrients you are depleting. It's pretty obvious that if you are going to deplete nutrients in the body, you are going to lose some sort of function in the body.

4) There is a wide variety of herbs and foods that can help thin the blood, such as:

a) Ginkgo, which is well known for thinning the blood and getting the blood to where it needs to go in the brain.

b) Garlic is well known for thinning the blood and helping the heart and the immune system.

5) Toxins like aluminum, found in everything from table salt to under arm deodorants, can slow down and/or shut off blood flow in these small capillaries depriving not only the brain but muscles and organs from the necessary oxygen.

a) Solution: Use rock salt with lots of alkalizing minerals rather than the detrimental table salt and make sure you use an antiperspirant that does not contain aluminum.

6) Avoid sugars:

Processed table sugars, high fructose corn syrups, etc. not only suppress the immune system but clump the red blood cells that deliver the oxygen. In order for the red blood cells to be able to uptake and release oxygen they have to be nice and circular and separated.

See:
http://www.wnho.net/soft_drinks_hard_facts.pdf

Increase plasticity in the arteries allowing for better blood flow and bringing down hypertension.

a) Solution: Increase Nitric Oxide which promotes vasodilatation by either increasing glutathione which regulates Nitric Oxide providing the body with the nutrients to make Nitric Oxide, or by eating healthy chocolate which:

i) Increases vasodilatation
ii) Reverses oxidized cholesterol
iii) Heals inflamed and ulcerated arteries
iv) There is currently so much on the internet about chocolate, just click and read. I always recommend Xocai™ chocolate as the best. Go to Appendix III to learn why.

Cancer cells have an incredible capacity to generate new blood vessels to gain access to greater amounts of nutrients. This is called angiogenesis.

a) Solution: We know of various foods and herbs that block this angiogenesis from happening. See Chapter 16, 17 & Appendix IV

Hypothyroid. Although this is a very misunderstood condition, what we want to look at is the amount of T3 in the body. While the thyroid produces T3 and T4 – T3 is by far more powerful. About 80% of the conversion of T4 to T3 occurs in the liver (if the liver is healthy and if the adrenals are not preventing it). Virtually every cell and every organ in the body requires T3. T3 is not only directly related to the metabolic process of every cell, increases the rate of protein synthesis, stimulates the breakdown of cholesterol, increases serotonin in the brain but it also directly increases blood flow.

See:

http://zimmer-foundation.org/sch/ajb.html

FOURTEEN

Research and alternatives treatments

How many research labs, scientific peer re-viewed articles and books written do we need before the general public becomes aware of the huge amount of data behind alternative thera-pies?

The challenge to alternative practitioners is that people do not look into alternative thera-pies until they have exhausted all conventional methods of becoming well. By then it is often too late for them or for a loved one.

The physician drops the bomb, "you have can-cer", and the client goes into a state of shock. For far too many, the belief is that the physi-cian has all the latest up-to-date answers and so, in a state of fear and ignorance of alterna-tives, the patient goes into a treatment program that is dangerous, toxic and too often ultimate-ly ends in death.

The following several chapters are going to address a number of different factors – each with a number of variables.

Read through the information then determine what you resonates with you. Go find a good health practitioner who will guide you through your healing journey.

The following chapters will cover:

- Essential Oils
- Organic Foods
- Herbs and their functions
- Herb salves
- Supplements
- Teas
- Tinctures
- Alkaline water, food, supplements.

Then we will look at some different modalities like:

- Ayurvedic
- Traditional Chinese Medicine
- German New Medicine

Please read on.

FIFTEEN

Organic Essential Oils

Dr. G. Young, ND includes essential oils in his cancer program claiming:

"Essential oils are some of the most concentrated natural extracts known, exerting significant antiviral, anti-inflammatory, antibacterial, hormonal, and psychological effects. Essential oils have the ability to penetrate cell membranes, travel throughout the blood and tissues, and enhance electrical frequencies. As we watch an essential oil work, it becomes clear that the powerful life force inherent in many essential oils gives them an unmatched ability to communicate and interact with cells in the human body."
(Dr. D Gary Young, Essential Oils Desk Reference, 2002).

Different oils are used for different cancers. Not all oils can be taken orally; some have to be applied topically. Others cannot be utilized in combination. Therefore, it is always important to get the advice of a trained and experienced practitioner. For example, lavender and frankincense are often used for breast cancers.

If you use a high-grade organic, quality lavender oil correctly, you will gain the following benefits:

1. Kills fungus, bacteria, and viruses, (major contributors to cancer).
2. Often used in perfume, due to its pleasing smell.
3. Helps treat anxiety, depression, nervous tension, and emotional stress.
4. Helps resolve various respiratory (lung) disorders. This could help with oxygen absorption in the lungs.
5. Helps improve blood circulation.
6. Immune system enhancement.
7. An excellent remedy for various types of pain.

SIXTEEN

Organic Food

If we go back to what Hippocrates, the father of Western Medicine, said, "Let food be thy medicine, and medicine be thy food" then it would appear that our bodies were designed to make use of the foods and herbs around us to grow, develop, maintain and heal. Whether you believe that we evolved or we were created or a combination of both – the same logic applies.

First, we will look at whole foods and then we will look at specific molecules in foods and what they do have to do with cancer.

Raw Organic Food

There has been a big push for raw food diets in the last couple of years. There are a lot of pros and cons to the raw food diet program. For instance, whole organic food that man has not got involved in changing is definitely preferable. In alternative medicine, there is a useful saying that goes like this: "The more man gets involved in the food process, the more detrimental the food is to the body."

In fact, the United States is one of the most overfed yet undernourished countries, not only in the world but throughout history. Unfortunately, Canada comes in at a close second.

Therefore, I'm sure most will agree that eating a whole food diet is of utmost importance.

Whole real organic foods, like we were designed to eat, have the vitamins, minerals, polyphenols, fatty acids, amino acids, antioxidants, etc. that our bodies require to create and maintain health.

These foods interact with our bodies so that we can make the over 10,000 enzymes, over 100 hormones, over 50 neurotransmitters, 29 collagens and all the different types of immune cells that our body requires to function effectively.

The challenges with the raw food diet are:

1. If a body already has cancer, the body is compromised. Therefore:
   a. Does the body have the enzymes to metabolize the food?
   b. Are the transport systems available to absorb the food from the gut into the blood and from the blood through the liver?

Consider these facts:

Steamed foods provoke activity in the food enzymes to help with the metabolic processes.

Some foods are better for us cooked, for instance, we have better access to the nutrients in tomatoes when they are cooked. We do not have the enzymes to break down the cellular structure in tomatoes in order to get the nutrient when eaten raw.

Raw foods are cold. In both Ayurvedic and Traditional Chinese medicine, cold, damp foods are not good for cancer. People trained in Traditional Chinese Medicine would say that a raw diet would create cold and damp congestion in the stomach/spline meridian. This is not considered to be a good thing.

Some people claim that if you add "hot and spicy" herbs you eliminate the concerns with a raw food diet. The opposing argument is that the "heating" herbs increase blood flow and metabolism but you want the body to put all of its energy into healing not be wasted heating foods to the temperature of the body.

So the easy solution is to steam your foods. Get the enzymes going, get the heat up but protect all the nutrients. This way, the body is not further burdened by heating the foods and the enzymes help metabolize the foods. That is a lot easier on a body that is already compromised.

Let's now look at some of the food molecules we want to have in our diet, that relate specifically to cancer.

There are a variety of molecules in our foods that work against cancer in a variety of ways. Each molecule will have a couple of sample medical articles to support their use in dealing with cancer.

1) **Betalaines** - Betalaines are the pigment coloration found in beets and prickly pear (72 types of betalaines; 24 categories) defined as:

   a. Phenolic composition, antioxidant capacity and in vitro cancer cell cytotoxicity of nine prickly pear (Opuntia spp.) juices.Chavez-Santoscoy RA, Gutierrez-Uribe JA, Serna-Saldívar SO. Source: Departamento de Biotecnología e Ingeniería de Alimentos, Tecnológico de Monterrey, Av. Eugenio Garza Sada 2501 Sur, Monterrey CP 64849, NL, México.

See:
http://www.ncbi.nlm.nih.gov/p
ubmed/19468836:

b. A study performed at the Department of Microbial Biosynthesis and Biotechnologies at The Stephan Angeloff Institute of Microbiology in Bulgaria revealed that betalaines possess antioxidant, anti-inflammatory, hepatoprotective and anti-cancer properties.

See:
http://www.livestrong.com/arti
cle/328258-what-are-the-benefits-
of-beet-root-vitamin-
supplements/#ixzz1zVnFoWZF

During the inflammatory process a chemical is released known as myeloperoxidase (MPE).

This is the most powerful oxidant produced by the human neutrophil during acute inflammation, especially from infection or cancer. Betalaines found in the Nopal cactus fruit extinguish the fire of inflammation caused by MPE and protect the healthy cells. Betalaines rescue the cell by quenching the fire of free radicals.

See:
http://thejuicynews.com/index.php/in
formation-and-betalains-
technical/information-and-betalains-
technical/

Beets also have betalaines, in fact, when
I had my cancer, my osteo-
path/naturopath told me to go on a
betalaine diet utilizing beets – the root
and leaf, pickled, baked, boiled, salad,
etc. The tumor was gone in three and
half weeks.

The betalaines found in beets not only
provide some cancer prevention capacity, especially against colon cancer but
also provide anti-oxidant, anti-
inflammatory and detoxing capacity. In
vitro (test tube or petri dish) lab tests
have reported beet betalaine suppression of human cancer cells.

Because different cancers evolve differently in response to the available nutrients and enzymes in a given place and
because of the type of genetic disorder
involved in the cell, the same remedy
does not work across all the different
types of cancers. Don't make the mis-

take of assuming that because this worked for one person, it should work for you.

2) Limonoids

Limonoids are molecules found in lemons, limes, citrus.
a) Limonoids inhibit tumor formation by promoting the formation of a detoxifying enzyme.
b) "Limonoids cause apoptosis (death) in cancer cells."

http://www.thebatt.com/2.8485/a-m-professor-focuses-on-citrus-for-cancer...

3) Polysaccharides

Not all polysaccharides are the same. The type we are referring to here are called beta glycan. Beta glycan are long chain polysaccharides and the most potent immuno-potentiating. Found in certain mushrooms, they can increase Natural Killer cells (a.k.a. NK) up to 3000%. NKs are a type of white blood cell that contributes to the immune system. They are anti-tumor cells.

These beta glycan are typically found in

mushrooms but not the typical store-bought mushrooms, which, by the way, have no nutrient value. Rather, beta glycan are found in mushrooms like the Agaricus Blazei Murrill mushroom, Cordyceps, Coriolus Veriscolor, Ganoderma Lucidum, Maitake Red Reishi and Shiitake.

a) Dr. Shoji Shibata, University of Tokyo, compared various different well-known cancer fighting and immune boosting mushrooms. He found that the Agaricus Blazei Murrill was the most potent of all the mushrooms, probably because they have the highest concentration of beta glycan.

Compared to other edible medicinal mushrooms, Agaricus Blazei Murrill was found to contain the highest concentration of polysaccharides, Beta 1, 3-D Glycan, Beta 1, 6-D Glycan, ergo sterols, linoleic acid, palmitorenic acid, Vitamin B6 and Vitamin B12.

b) Dr. Shoji Shibata, a professor from the Pharmacological department of Tokyo University, and Dr. Ikegawa, a physician from the Japan National Cancer Centre, researched the ABM mushroom. The research focused on the anti-tumor properties of the Beta Glycan polysaccharides found in Agaricus Blazei Murrill, (over 30 years ago).

See:
http://www.shikoku.ne.jp/ys/blaz
ei.html
sekkei@ys.shikoku.ne.jp

c) Research papers regarding beta glycan found in Agaricus Blazei Murrill and their effectiveness against breast cancer, colon cancer, liver cancer, lung cancer and ovarian cancer were presented to the Japan Cancer Society, 1980.

d) Dr. Mamdooh Ghneum, King Drew Medical Centre of UCLA reported that the Agaricus Blazei Murrill beta glycan not only increased the number of Natural Killer cells (NK) but also made each individual cell more powerful. He presented his findings to the 9th World Immunology Congress held in San Francisco, 1995.

See:
www.bioresis.com/mushroom_god.
html

e)http://www.betaglucan.org/histo
ry.htm identifies a number of universities, researchers, and papers of
those who have researched beta glycan and cancer.

f) "Beta glycan" refers generally, but
not always, to Beta- 1,3/1,6-glucan.
"Scleroglucan" and "PSAT" are two
Beta-1, 3/1, 6-polysaccharides. Beta
glycan are derived primarily from
yeast cell wall, various fungi, grains,
and mushrooms. Beta 1, 4 glucan is
derived from oats and barley, mini-
mally effective in immune potentiation and not included in this research summary of forms of Beta
1,3/1,6 glycan. Many beta glycan are
marketed under various trademark
names that are not unique ingredi-
ent formulations.

See:
http://www.ncbi.nlm.nih.gov/pub
med/19468836

g) Beta 1,3-D Glycan works by acti-
vating the macrophages, or immune

cells which trap and engulf foreign substances. These activated cells start a cascade of events that cause the entire system to be alerted and mobilized in an entirely naturally activated sequence. This amplified immune system response helps speed up the recovery of damaged tissue, helps other substances like antibiotics, anti-fungals and anti-parasitic to work better, and helps the macrophages recognize and destroy mutated cells.

See:
http://www.greenehaven.com/Bet a.html#summary

(Why doesn't your oncologist know about all these studies?)

4) Procyanidins

Another nutrient found in foods, like chocolate, apples, grape seed.

Procyanidins also promote apoptosis (or death) in cancer cells. In fact, there is a large amount of these anti-oxidants found in chocolate that has a special patent that protects its anti-oxidants, i.e., Xocai chocolate (see Appendix III)

a) Chemo preventive properties of apple procyanidins on human colon cancer-derived metastatic SW620 cells and in a rat model of colon carcinogenesis: Francine Gossé1, Sylvain Guyot2, Stamatiki Roussi1, Annelise Lobstein3, Barbara Fischer1, Nikolaus Seiler1 and Francis Raul1,*+ Author Affiliations

See: http://carcin.oxfordjournals.org/content/early/2005/.../carcin.bgi074.full.pd.

b) Procyanidins inhibit proliferation (tumor growth) and promote apoptosis of the prostate cancer cell line LNCaP. [Article in Chinese] Wu ZQ, Huang H, Ding XM, Luo RC. Source: Department of Oncology, Nanfang Hospital, Southern Medical University, Guangzhou. Procyanidins can also effect : intracellular signaling pathways, or communication between cells; synthesis of polyamines, or compounds that include more than two primary amino acids (proteins); and trigger apoptosis in tumor cells, or preprogrammed cell death.

These compounds antagonize cancer promotion in vivo. In contrast with absorbable drugs, these natural, non-toxic, dietary constituents reach the colon where they are able to exert their anti-tumor effects.

See:
http://carcin.oxfordjournals.org/content/26/7/1291.ful

c) Skin cancer – grape seed proanthocyanidins decreased tumor numbers and reduced the malignancy of papillomas.

See:
http://en.wikipedia.org/wiki/Grape_seed_extract

Again, why doesn't your oncologist know about all of this if the goal is to heal or prevent cancer?

SEVENTEEN

Herbs

It is interesting to look at the research and find that allopathic medications are made from molecules and nutrients from herbs and plants. The challenge is that when the individual molecule is isolated and synthesized and made in a laboratory, these artificial substitutions typically do more harm than good. Take a look at the following examples:

1. Periwinkle, or Vinca rosea linn. This herb was redesigned into Vincristine sulfate which can cause severe skin damage, nerve damage and loss of various sensations and senses.

   In its natural form vinblastine and vincristine are very important cancer fight molecules which have been known to increase survival of childhood leukemia from 10% to 95%! (and used to treat Hodgkin's Disease).

   See:
   http://www.livingrainforest.org/about-rainforests/anti-cancer-rosy-

periwinkle.

See:
http://web.mit.edu/newsoffice/2006/
periwinkle-1115.html

2. Vinca rosea also became Vinblastine sulfate which causes damage to white
   blood cells along with hair loss, nausea,
   constipation, and can lead to hepatitis.

3. A molecule from the Yew tree, paclitax-
   el, was isolated and synthesized and became the drug called Taxol – which
   causes nerve damage, depletion of neutrophils, hair loss, nausea, vomiting, inflammation of mucous membranes,
   muscle pain, and venous inflammation.
   Before man got involved, however, it
   was very effective.

   See:
   http://www.whale.to/w/orthodox_her
   bs.html\

Numerous herbs are known for a variety of
different effects on cancer. One has to be very
careful when designing a particular herbal
remedy for cancer. There are lots of different
factors to take into consideration:

1. Do the herbs work synergistically together?

2. Are the herbs neurotoxic or cardio toxic, either on their own or when combined?

3. What herbs work with what cancers?

4. Are the nutrients in the herbs feeding the patient or feeding the cancer?

5. What is the most effective way to taking the herb?

   a. tincture

   b. topically

   c. capsule

   d. food

6. Also what specific species is being utilized? Where was the herb grown? When and how was it harvested and what processing did it encounter? All these considerations have an impact on the benefit of the herb.

7. Unless one is a well-trained herbalist, one should not play with these variables.

8. Always find a good, trained health practitioner with whom to work.

One of my supervisors while doing my herbal training had not only worked predominantly with cancer patients but had written books and taught at the Mayo Clinic. This doctor's success rate with healing cancers varied in the 90th percentile. I don't know of one oncologist who could beat that.

The following herbs are ones that are known to destroy tumors. There are a number of ways these herbs can functions and so they have been organized according the mechanistic action that utilize to destroy tumors.

1. **DISCUTIENTS** – Dissolve and remove tumors and other abnormal growths.
    a. Burdock root (Arctium lappa)
    b. Chaparral (Larrea tridentate)
    c. Garlic (Allium sativum)
    d. Red clover tops (Trifolium pretense)
    e. Sorrel (Rumex acetosa)
    f. Tumeric (Curcuma longa)

2. **ALKALIZING** – As mentioned earlier, cancers thrive in acidic environments and even create their own acidic environment. So if we can include herbs that help to alkalize the system, that is another factor in working with the cancer cells. We look to herbs that are full of calcium, magnesium, oxygen, potassium, selenium, zinc and Vitamins B and C, such as:

a. Dandelion greens (Taraxacum off.)
b. Garlic (Allium sativum)
c. Stinging Nettles (Urtica diocia
d. Turmeric (Curcuma longa)
e. Wheat grass (Triticum asetivum)

3. **ALTERATIVES** – These herbs are great for both the blood and the lymph system by cleansing the system and making it easier for the body to eliminate the cancer cells. One can clean the blood and the lymph system by addressing the liver and intestines primarily but also but cleaning the kidneys and spleen.

Cancer patients are typically in a weakened state so this type of cleansing/detoxing needs to be done gently and effectively.

- Barberry (Berberis)
- Burdock root (Articum lappa)

Cayenne - Dr. Schulze's mentor, Dr. John Christopher, stated that "We can do wonderful things with cayenne we are not able to do with any other known herb," while Dr. Schulze agrees that, "There is no other herb that increases your blood flow faster than cayenne. There are none that work faster; none that work better." It is truly an amazing herb. (David Tanton, <u>Taking The Mystery out of Cancer</u>, 2011, p. 108)

- Chaparral (Larrea tridentate)
- Chickweed (Stellaria media)
- Cleavers (Galium aparine)
- Comfrey (Symphytum off.)
- Dandelion (Taraxacum off.)
- Echinacea (Echinacea agustifolia)
- Garlic (Allium sativum)
- Ginseng (Elethrococus)
- Goldenseal (Hydrastis Canadensis)
- Gotu kola (Centella asiatica)
- Licorice root (Glycyrryhiza)
- Oregon grape root (Mahonia aquifolium)
- Poke root (Phytolacca)
- Prickly ash (Zanthoxylum)
- Red clover tops (Trifolium pretense)
- Rhubarb (Rheum rhaponticum)
- Sassafras (sassafras albidum)
- Yellow dock (Rumex crispus)

4. **ANTIBIOTICS**: Because the immune system is already weakened with the cancer, the body will be more susceptible to various viruses and bacteria. These are some herbs that inhibit the

growth of, and destroy, viruses and bacteria, and strengthen the body's immune system.

- Chaparral (Larrea tridentate)
- Echinacea (Echinacea agustifolia)
- Garlic (Allium sativum)
- Goldenseal (Hydrastis Canadensis)

4a) ANTISEPTICS: These herbs do not kill bacteria but rather prevent the growth of bacteria. So again they can be helpful to a weakened immune system.

- Barberry (Berberis)
- Echinacea (Echinacea agustifolia)
- Garlic (Allium sativum)
- Goldenseal (Hydrastis Canadensis)

4b) IMMUNE BOOSTERS: Because the immune system is weak, we can also provide herbs that strengthen the immune system.

- Astragalus (Astragalus membranaceus)
- Echinacea (Echinacea agustifolia)
- Ginseng Elethrococus, Panax, Red

- Mistletoe (Viscum album)

5. **ANTI-OXIDANTS** – These molecules neutralize free radicals. While our bodies utilize free radicals in certain situations, for instance the immune system, by and large we have way too many free radicals in our bodies because of lifestyle, diet and stress. These free radicals are produced in our bodies naturally as a result of any enzyme process but they are also contributed to with:

- Pesticides

- Herbicides

- Metal toxicity

- Low levels of glutathione

- Medications

- Over exposure to the sun with the use of sunscreens that are full of carcinogens and protect us from the UVB rays rather than the UVA rays

- Toxins in our cleaning products

- Toxins in our hygiene and make up products

- Extensive exercise, ie., cardio exercise

- All the issues that deplete our glutathione – see Chapter 18

Solution: Increase anti-oxidants in both our foods and herbs.

a. Foods

    i. Xocai® chocolate – properly processed to keep all the anti-oxidants – 3 pieces = 12 servings of fruits and vegetables in anti-oxidants alone (over 300 nutrients important to the body)

    ii. Acai berry – if properly processed

    iii. Blueberries

    iv. Mangosteen

    v. Pecans

    vi. Elderberry

    vii. Pomegranate

    viii. Cranberries

b. Herbs

    i. Rhodolia rosea

    ii. Cloves, Cinnamon, Cardamom

iii. Turmeric, Ginger
iv. Oregano, Sage, Thyme

6. **HEPATICS** – As noted in other chapters, when dealing with cancers you always have to look after the liver. We need to look at herbs that are particularly good for the liver, detoxing, strengthening, and protecting the liver and promoting bile.

When the cleansing occurs too fast (which can easily happen if the diet and herbal formula is correct), the liver can become overloaded and stop functioning. This is called hepatic coma and death results.

6a) CHOLAGOGUES – these are medicinal agents that promote the discharge of bile from the liver to the gallbladder and on to the intestine.

a) Barberry (Berberis)
b) Cayenne (Capsicum)
c) Dandelion (Taraxacum off)
d) Goldenseal (Hydrastis Canadensis)
e) Yellow dock (Rumex crispus)

6b) HEPATICS – As opposed to detoxifying the liver by creating more bile, these are herbs, which strengthen, tone, and stimulate the secretive functions of the liver.

- Aloe vera
- Barberry (Berberis)
-

6c) LIVER TONICS – Herbs increase the energy of the liver.

- Barberry
- Buckthorn bark (Rhamus purshiana)
- Cleavers (Trifolium pretense)
- Mistletoe (Viscum album)

6d) GALLBLADDER TONICS – Herbs strengthen the gallbladder, where the bile from the liver is produced.

- Goldenseal (Hydrastis Canadensis)
- Oregon grape root (Mahonia aquifolium)

7. **INTESTINAL TONICS** – A strong intestinal tract is always required. This is where the body decides what to absorb and what to eliminate. We need a healthy flora of bacteria that aid the process of digestion and metabolizing

nutrients that we require.
- Barberry (Berberis)
- Goldenseal (Hydrastis Canaden-
sis)
- Rhubarb (Rheum rhaponticum)

8. **KIDNEY TONICS** – The kidneys are
important because they filter the blood.
They make your urine and enable the
body to get rid of toxins. These herbs
strengthen the kidneys.

- Burdock root (Rhamus purshi-
ana)
- Cleavers (Trifolium pretense)
- Mistletoe (Viscum album)

9. **LYMPHATICS** – The lymph system is
often referred to as the sewage system.
Excess cellular "stuff" and toxins and
byproducts are dumped into the lymph
system. This system tries to work the
molecules so that they won't harm the
blood. They attempt to keep the blood
clean.

- Chaparral (Larrea tridentate)
- Dandelion (Taraxacum off)
- Echinacea (Echinacea augus-
tofolia)
- Garlic (Allium sativum)

- Oregon grape root (Mahonia aquifolium)
- Poke root (Phytolacca)
- Yellow dock (Rumex crispus)

10. **MUCILAGES** – Often times as the body is ridding itself of the toxins, the mucilage gets harmed. Mucilage is the mucus membrane that lines the intestinal track out through the rectum, the mouth and nose, and down through the respiratory tract in the body. These are herbs that tend to soothe inflamed parts. Slippery elm is the best of them.

- Chickweed (Stellaria media)
- Comfrey (Symphytum off.)
- Slippery elm (Ulmdus rubra)

Often there is pain with cancer yet cancer itself does not cause pain. The pain can be stimulated through different pathways. So, while we can provide herbs for pain, the practitioner needs to know why the pain pathways are being stimulated.

Increased levels of toxicity, especially in the later stages of cancer, tends to cause the pain. The liver, kidneys and bowels need to get rid of these toxins – or pain can result.

As mentioned in the section under Teas, the Gerson Institute, utilized coffee enemas to help get the toxin out of the rectum.

11. **NERVINES** – While there are a number of nervine herbs, if the pain is due to toxic overload, the nervines are not likely to help.

- Chamomile (Matricaria recutita)
- Mistletoe (Viscum album)
- Gravel root (Eutrochium)

12. **ANODYNES** – Again, these relieve pain but by decreasing reaction in the nerves and nerve centers.

13. **ANTI-SPASMODIC** (antiparalysis) – Function in a similar way to anodynes.

- Echinacea
- White willow

The following is a more detailed explanation of some specific herbs:
1) Ashwagandha: (Withania somnifera)

A well-known Ayurvedic herb used in India, home of Ayurvedic medicine, historically, Ashwagandha has been medicinally utilized for fatigue, dehydration, bone weakness, anti-aging, restoring memory loss and cell destruction. Recently, however, Wadhwa and Kaul from the National Institute of Advanced Industrial Science and Technology, Japan, also recognized Ashwagandha as anti-carcinogenic. Like many other plants, it has the intelligence to kill the cancerous cells while leaving the healthy cells alone.

They stated: "Most cancer cells occur due to aging and when loss of cell equilibrium occurs. With Ashwagandha possessing anti-aging and anti-cancer properties, the uneven multiplication of cells is also slowed down which protects the body from cancer." Their studies have been published in Clinical Cancer Research, Plos One, Journal of Gerontology – all US journals.

See:

http://www.biotechmashup.com/beta/Biotechnoloy/Selective_Killing_of_Cancer_Cells_by_Ashwagadha_Leaf_Extract_and_Its_Compone nt_Withanone_Involves_ROS_Signaling-1/related_links

http://science.lecture.ub.ac.id/publications/

In addition, Ashwagandha has also been

shown to protect from some of the damages done by chemotherapy. Chemotherapy can cause neutropenia or a decrease in neutrophils, a white blood cell that comprises part of the immune system. This is partly why chemotherapy patients are vulnerable to infection. Ashwagandha extract protects the body from this decrease in neutrophils.

(Indian Journal of Physiology and Pharmacology, 2001, Vol. 45, Issue 2, pp. 253-257)

Natural food and herb sources of Lithium can also help increase neutrophils. For instance, the nightshade vegetables like potatoes, peppers, and tomatoes, plus grains or herbs like chamomile.

2. Mistletoe extract: (Viscum album)

European mistletoe extract has been shown to kill cancer cells in the laboratory as well as to stimulate the immune system. Three components of mistletoe are thought to be of particular use – lectins, alkaloids and viscotoxins. They are usually injected subcutaneously, ideally near the tumor. However, sometimes it has been injected directly into the tumor.

See:
http://www.biomedcentral.com/14712407/9/451

http://www.cancer.gov/cancertopics/pdq/cam/mistletoe/patient/page2

3. Red Clover (Trifolium pretense) – Well-known for skin cancers.

Red Clover (one of the ingredients of his cancer poultice) is famous for resolving skin cancer, a specific for melanoma. I have had patients kill and lift off melanomas like a scab, flaking off a wound that has healed. I had one lady with a severe melanoma on her left arm. The cancer was black in color and the blood in the arm was also infected...One doctor even suggested amputation...In a week's time half the cancer was gone...In 3 weeks her cancer was gone and never returned." Dr. Richard Shulze.

4. Turmeric, ginger = curcumin (Curcuma longa, Zingerberaceae)

Numerous studies have shown the benefits of turmeric over the past decade. However, this is not new. Ayurvedic and Traditional Chinese Medicines have known this for 1000s of years. As usual,

Western science is far behind. In some ways, we are just coming out of the dark ages.

One of the sought-after molecules in Turmeric is curcumin (likewise with ginger). Turmeric has a long list of properties, like anti-inflammatory, anti-oxidant, etc. but let's look at the ways it is involved with cancer cells.

a) Curcumin inhibits vascular epithelial growth factors. Cancer needs these growth factors in order to create new blood vessels. This process is called angiogenesis and allows the tumors to rob the body of more nutrients.

b) Curcumin kills B lymphoma cells.

c) Curcumin blocks the COX-2 enzyme that produces the negative inflammation which is a precursor to cancer.

d) Turmeric is a significant anti-inflammatory.

e) Works well with other anti-oxidants, ie., resveratrol and green tea's EGCG.

f) In addition, turmeric also inhibits "bad" bacteria in the stomach and the intestines.

g) Boosts glutathione levels – this is

extremely important, as we will
see under the section on Supplements.

h) Turmeric helps prevent liver damage.

i) Turmeric is involved in Oxygen homeo-
stasis.

j) Turmeric also turns on apoptosis, the
death of cancer cells.

k) Turmeric has enzymes of crucial
importance in the immune system.

l) Turmeric is involved in the metabolism
of essential fatty acid.

See:
http://www.canceractive.com/cancer-active-
page-link.aspx?n=1571

Professor Bharat Aqqarwal, Ph. D. in MD An-
derson's Department of Therapeutics, has con-
ducted a number of studies showing that in
pancreatic cancer patients having no chemotherapy, turmeric reduced tumor size. He believes it is effective against many types of cancer because it suppresses angiogenesis (the
growth of blood vessels essential to a tumor).

See:
http://www.canceractive.com/cancer-active-
page-link.aspx?n=1571

- Br J Clinical Pharmacology 1998

Jan;45(1):1-12; update Toxicol Lett 2000 Mar 15;112-113:499-505). They observed that curcumin slows the rate at which hormone-responsive prostate cancer cells become resistant to hormonal therapy.

- In Japan, researchers defined curcumin as a broad-spectrum anti-cancer agent: Iqbal M, et al. Pharmacol Toxicol. 2003 Jan, 92(1):33-8).
- Vimala, S., et al., Anti-tumor promoter activity in Malaysian ginger rhizobia used in traditional medicine. British Journal of Cancer, Vol. 80, No. 1/2, April 1999, pp. 110-16.

Herb salves for cancers

Dr. Richard Shulze Salve – Red Clover blossoms, Poke root, goldenseal, activated charcoal, Tea Tree Oil, Bentonite clay, Slippery Elm inner bark.

See:
http://www.whale.to/cancer/salves.html

Tincture

Herbal medicine utilizes tinctures that are typically an alcoholic extract of a plant or animal material. The alcohol may be anywhere between a 25 to a 90% proof. Although alcohol is by far the most common solvent, other solvents may involve vinegar, glycerol, and propylene glycols.

A herbal tincture for cancer may involve 5-7 herbs. Each herb will address a number of different issues so in combination you can address all the different issues identified under QUALITIES DESIRED IN A CANCER HERBAL FORMULA.

An example of a herbal tincture might be:

Hoxsey formula: Red clover, Burdock root, Barberry bark, Licorice root, Buckthorn bark, Prickly ash, poke berries and root, Stillingia root, Cascara amarga.

There are also a number of Chinese herb formulas that work well with cancers. See the section on Traditional Chinese Medicine for these various other healing responses.

See:
http://www.majidali.com/spice_medicine_and_oxygen_part_2.htm

EIGHTEEN

Supplements

1. Glutathione

What is glutathione? In its simplest form, it is called a tripeptide, a substance made up of three amino acids plus sulfur and thiol. Additionally, glutathione is a complex of enzymes, transferases, synthetase, reductase and more. Research shows that when one component is affected, they are all affected.

While under the heading of supplements, glutathione does not work as a supplement. The reason for this is that there are no transport mechanisms to get glutathione into the cell. There are a couple of places where glutathione is transported out of the cells, for instance in the liver and the kidneys, but we don't know of anywhere it gets transported into the cell.

Unfortunately, if we simply take glutathione as a supplement, it breaks down in the hydrochloric acid of the stomach and we lose the most vulnerable part, the cysteine.

Therefore, glutathione has to be made inside the cell. How can we make that happen?

We now have two ways we can do this. The first is to turn on the tools to make glutathione at a genetic level. Dr. McCord, an American biochemist and Nobel Prize winner, is the scientist who came up with a formula that does just that. Interestingly, the formula has both turmeric and ashwagandha in it. Given the properties of these two substances, this is not surprising.

Even more interesting is that this formula is being studied in more than 20 universities and with fantastic results.

The second method is to give the cell the "pancake mix" of all the right nutrients, in the right ratio, to make glutathione. Dr. Keller, a world-renowned physician/ scientist, who was an internist, oncologist and immunologist; and came up with that formula.

Both of these products are available to the public. See information on how to access them in Appendix III.

Now, let's look at what glutathione actually does. It is one of the most important molecules in the body.

i) Master Anti-oxidant – glutathione is claimed to be a million times more powerful than any anti-oxidant we can get from food or supplement.

- Endogenous – made inside of the cell
- Re-stabilizes itself and all other anti-oxidants
- Deals with all 6 categories of free radicals
- Works inside cell, in cell membrane and also outside of cell

ii) Detoxification

- Major component of Phase II in liver detox
- Major component of all cellular detoxification

iii) Chelator

- A chelator, in effect, attaches to the toxic metals and pulls them out of the body through the kidneys.

- Glutathione is well recognized as a very good chelator for most toxic metals so rather than having to utilize needles for a chelation therapy or takes various herbs or supplements, one just needs to increase his or her body's glutathione levels.

iv) Inflammation

- Major component of healthy inflammation resolution

v) Hormone regulation

- Involved either directly or indirectly with all hormones in the body

vi) Cellular Energy

- Cellular energy is provided by the ATP; created by the mitochondria – GSH is the only known molecule that protects the mitochondria

vii) Prostaglandin synthesis

- Vasodilation/constriction

viii) Nitric Oxide regulation

- Which regulates hormones, vasodilation, immune system,

ix) DNA

- Protects DNA from going sideways; involved in both repair and elimination of abnormal DNA
- also required in protein synthesis

x) Cellular transport

- Required for most amino acid transportation in the cells

xi) Anti-aging

- Involved, like other anti-oxidants, in preventing telomere breakdown but is also the only known molecule that can provoke telomere creation

xii) Calcium movement
- Required for regulation of Ca movement (gating of cardio cell function)

xiii) Respiratory

- 40% required in RBC to both pick up/release both O2 & CO2

xiv) Immune System

- Immune cells like, Lymphocytes, like T cells, B cells, macrophages, TNF, NK require, on average, about 62% to both develop and function
- In addition, glutathione regulates the balance between T1 and T2 cells – if either group is predominant; there is a whole group of dysfunctions, syndromes and diseases that can occur.

There are currently over 95,000 articles regarding glutathione, on a wide variety of topics. With regard to glutathione, most chemotherapy can be divided into two categories:

a) those that encourage glutathione (to eliminate the cancer)
b) those that try to eliminate glutathione (so that it doesn't try to eliminate the chemotherapy)

Here are a couple of scientific articles regarding glutathione and its role in cancer.

a) "With respect to cancer, glutathione metabolism is able to play both protective and pathogenic roles. It is crucial in the removal and detoxification of carcinogens, and alterations in this pathway can have a profound effect on cell survival. However, by conferring resistance to a number of chemotherapeutic drugs, elevated levels of glutathione in tumor cells are able to protect such cells in bone marrow, breast, colon, larynx and lung cancers. Here we present a number of studies investigating the role of glutathione in promoting cancer, impeding chemotherapy, and the use of glutathione modulation to enhance antineoplastic therapy."

See:
http://www.ncbi.nlm.nih.gov/pubmed/15386533

b) This article discusses the molecular epidemiology of the human glutathione Stransferase genotypes GSTM1 and GSTT1 in cancer susceptibility.

See:
http://cebp.aacrjournals.org/content/6/9/733.short

c) http://www.immune-health-solutions-for-you.com/glutathione-and-cancer.html

This article discusses how glutathione is both a preventative and a treatment.

2. Super Phytoplankton

Plankton has a molecular structure that is similar to red blood cells but our bodies cannot tell the difference between the plankton and a red blood cell. Because they carry oxygen they can provide the oxygen that the body is lacking in due to anemias, cancer and other conditions.
There is a variety of different types of plankton people can utilize, so make sure you have a good health practitioner who can direct you to a good product.

3. CoQ10

CoQ10 is an important molecule to every cell in the body. As mentioned earlier, most enzyme processes in every cell require ATP, the necessary cellular fuel, in order to function. CoQ10 is the limiting factor in making the ATP.

What is a limiting factor? If I asked you to make pancakes for a one hundred people and you had an unlimited supply of flour, milk, and baking powder but only one egg – the one egg would be your limiting factor. That is what CoQ10 is when the cells are making ATP.

In every cell, there are organs (called organelles in a cell). One of the organelles is called the mitochondria. It is the mitochondria that make the ATP fuel. How many mitochondria a given cell will have will be entirely dependent on the amount of fuel the cell requires. For example, a heart cell that has to continually function, night and day. We really don't want it to stop so it will have upwards of a 1,000 mitochondria in any given cell.

(As a side note, the statin drugs that block the liver from making the cholesterol that is required for so many different functions in the body and is the precursor to a whole number of other molecules, also block the body's capacity to make CoQ10.)

This fact has been known for decades in Europe. In fact, for some twenty-five years, drug companies were not allowed to make statin drugs without sufficient CoQ10 to compensate for what the statin drug was depleting. That knowledge has only just recently been leaking into the minds of cardiac medical professionals in North America, yet it is the same pharmaceutical companies that make the statin drugs in both places. Why is that?

Currently, there is controversy over which type of CoQ10 is more effective and for what age group. Make sure you check with your Health Practitioner to determine which kind is best for you, or do some of your own research and become informed for the sake of your own health.

4. Iodine

Numerous conditions are associated with iodine deficiencies, the main one of which is hypothyroid. Iodine is necessary to create both T4 and T3. While T3 is 4 times more powerful than T4 – your body makes 4 times more T4. Thus we need to convert the T4 to T3 and this conversion happens mostly in the liver – another reason to keep the liver functioning well.

The fluoride in anti-depressants like Prozac can actually deplete iodine levels. So, if your depression was initially due to a hypothyroid condition, taking an anti-depressant will actually make the condition even worse.

Further, hypothyroid is known to increase the risk of cancer. Most people are familiar with the thyroid needing iodine to make T3 and T4 and that T3 and T4 are required by virtually every cell in the body. They are involved in the following processes:

- Energy (the mitochondria which produce the ATP fuel are dependent on T3 to function).

- Vasodilation of the arteries (T3 stimulates the synthesis of, secretion of, and action of vasodilators).

- Regulates body temperature (over 3000 enzymes are dependent on the appropriate body temperature).

- Regulates control of cholesterol breakdown in the liver.

- Regulates body weight – increase or expenditure of energy/metabolism.

- Regulates sensitivity to various hormones, like adrenaline, causing passive depression at one end and agitated depression and anxiety at the other end.

- Involved in growth hormone (in

the brain and throughout the body).

- Brain function – involved in the ability to both lay down new neural patterns (learning) as well as maintaining old pathways.

- Reproduction - involved in the synthesis and release of reproductive hormones from the pituitary gland.

- Involved in the regulation of your heart rate – perhaps excess T3 increases sensitivity to adrenaline – therefore the heart will beat faster.

- Regulates the speed of hair, nails, and skin growth.

- Involved in the function of insulin itself as well as other components of the blood-glucose process starting with the liver.

See:
http://suite101.com/article/understanding-the-t3-and-t4-thyroid-hormones-a134923

http://www.ncbi.nlm.nih.gov/pubmed/12714012

http://www.ncbi.nlm.nih.gov/pubmed/3781233

In fact, the thyroid requires approximately 6mg/day of iodine but we need iodine for more than T4 & T4. For instance, the breasts require another 5mg/day of iodine. The rest of the body requires about 2 mg/day. Unfortunately, the RDA (Note: The RDA levels for almost every nutrient have been long recognized as insufficient.) says that we only need 150mcg/day.

Iodine acts as an anti-bacterial molecule, which is why it is used as a skin disinfectant and also used in water purification systems.
In addition, iodine helps prevent fibrocystic breast disease by modulating estrogen in breast tissue.

The challenge is that if a physician prescribes for hypothyroid the drug of choice will probably be Synthroid, which has a good probability of creating rT3. The subject of the thyroid is immense enough to require its own book however, suffice to say that T4 and T3 are required for cellular functioning and when they are disrupted, we have a higher risk of cancer...so we need to resolve the problem not just manage the symptoms.

Iodine deficiency has been associated with the following:

- Fibrocystic breast disease
- Breast cancer
- Fibromyalgia
- Chronic Fatigue syndrome
- Ovarian cancer
- Uterine fibroid tumors
- Thyroid problems (almost all of them)
- Fungal infections
- Bronchial asthma
- COPD
- Cretinism
- Fluoride, bromide and chloride toxicity

See:
http://www.bartonpublishing.com/blog/iodine-cancer-cure/

Foods rich in iodine are:

- Cranberries
- Graviola (Soursop)
- Mineral salts
- Organic potatoes

- Organic navy beans
- Organic strawberries
- Organic yogurt
- Sea vegetables

5. Vitamin C

Unfortunately, Vitamin C is a much misunderstood vitamin even though it is vitally important.

Vitamin C bought in a health food store is typically a synthetic version and is simply a replicate of the most outer ring of the whole Vitamin C molecule.
Vitamin C moves into six different structures in the body. Each structure is responsible for different functions. Dr. Ben Kin, a Canadian chiropractor and researcher, claims that the whole Vitamin C is a complex molecule made up of:

- Rutin
- Bioflavonoids (vitamin P)
- Factor K
- Factor J
- Factor P

- Tyrosinase

- Ascorbinogen

- Ascorbic Acid

See:
http://choicesunlimited.ca/content/difference
-between-ascorbic-acid-and-real-vitamin-c

This outer ring of Vitamin C does function as an anti-oxidant but only if the pH of the body is above 7.4. Remember, cancer patients typically have a very low acidic pH.

In order to get the real benefit from Vitamin C you need the whole molecule, not a manufactured synthetic product. The whole vitamin is additionally involved in the following:

- Helps to form collagen, which is a key structural component of your bones, ligaments, tendons, and blood vessels.

- Acts as a powerful antioxidant, protecting your cells against damage and premature aging due to free radicals, toxins, and other harmful substances that make their way into your blood.

- Prevents damage to fatty acids, amino acids and glucose in your blood.

- Helps to make norepinephrine, a hormone that is essential to the health of your nervous system.

See:
http://choicesunlimited.ca/content/difference
-between-ascorbic-acid-and-real-vitamin-c

When it comes to cancer, Vitamin C interacts with various metals, like iron, and creates hydrogen peroxide. Hydrogen peroxide is important to the immune system and functions as a signaling molecule calling white blood cells to injured areas requiring attention.

Hydrogen peroxide is also believed to destroy the mitochondria and DNA of cells with altered DNA, i.e., cancer cells.

Good food sources for Vitamin C include:

Whole-Food Sources	Serving	Vitamin C (mg)
Sweet red pepper	1/2 cup, raw	141
Strawberries	1 cup	82
Orange	1 medium	70
Brussels sprouts	1/2 cup	68
Broccoli, cooked	1/2 cup	58
Collard greens, cooked	1/2 cup	44
Grapefruit	1/2 med.	44

Cantaloupe	1/4 med.	32
Cabbage, cooked	1/2 cup	24
Tomato	1 medium	23

See:
http://www.DrBenKim.com

Be careful not to try to utilize fruit juices for Vitamin C as they have lost all of their skin, lining and seeds. This leaves predominantly the sugars, which will feed the cancer. When you utilize fruits, make sure you eat the whole fruit and get all the fiber, minerals and nutrients in the skin, lining and flesh.

Also beware that fruit juice is not combined with sodium benzoates. Independently, the two cause no problem for the body but combined, they form a benzene carcinogen. This benzene has been found in 54 of the 84 soft drinks tested by the FDA but no one seems to have heard anything about it.

6. Vitamin D3

Although it is really a hormone, Vitamin D3 is an important molecule to the body. Dr. Mercola's website has a wide number of articles for simple reading with regard to all the benefits of Vitamin D.

Top 10 facts about vitamin D and cancer:

1. Many studies have found solar ultraviolet-B (UVB) Vitamin D associated with reduced risk of breast, colon and rectal cancer.

2. A randomized controlled trial with 1100 IU/day Vitamin D3 plus 1450 mg/day calcium found a 77% reduction in all cancer incidence.

3. Geographical studies have found reduced risk in mortality rates for 15-20 types of cancer in regions of higher solar UVB doses.

4. Observational studies found risk of breast, colon, and rectal cancer falls as Vitamin D blood levels rise to over 40 ng/mL (100 nmol/L).

5. Mechanisms have been proposed to explain how Vitamin D acts to reduce the risk of cancer from starting, growing, and spreading.

6. Those who develop non-melanoma skin cancer may have produced enough Vitamin D to reduce their risk of internal cancers.

7. Those with higher Vitamin D blood levels at time of cancer diagnosis had nearly twice the survival rate of those with the lowest levels.

8. African-Americans have an increased

risk of cancer in part due to lower Vitamin D blood levels because of darker skin.

9. Higher UVB exposure early in life has been found associated with reduced risk of breast and prostate cancer.

10. Those diagnosed with breast, colon and prostate cancer in summer in Norway had higher survival rates than those diagnosed in winter.

See:
http://www.vitamindcouncil.org/health-conditions/cancer/

In all, we have identified 89 studies that describe how greater Vitamin D levels reduce cancers of the breast, prostate, colon, esophagus, pancreas, ovary, rectum, bladder, kidney, lung and uterus, as well as Non-Hodgkin's lymphoma and multiple myeloma. Vitamin D has an effect on at least 200 human genes. Many of these genes are responsible for regulating cell proliferation, differentiation, and apoptosis.

Proliferation is uncontrolled cell division (cancer cells are characterized by rapid and uncontrolled division).

Differentiation is the process that cells undergo

to mature into normal cells (uncontrolled re-production of immature [undifferentiated] cells is a defining feature of cancer).

Apoptosis is the natural termination of defective cells (cancer cells are resistant to natural destruction making them difficult to eradicate).

(Tanton, Taking the Mystery out of Cancer, 2011, p.192)

Other supplements:

The body is a phenomenally interactive and dynamic system. There is a massive number of molecules that are going to have an effect somewhere, somehow in the body.
Different supplements will have a different impact in different pathways that prevent and/or stop cancers in a wide variety of ways.
This is why it is important to work with some-one who understands your body and your can-cer to help you design a protocol that works with your system.

It is also important to recognize and under-stand that cancers can change their DNA to ac-commodate what you are doing so you need to keep changing the protocol until you bring your body into its optimal healing process.

This is why it is so important not to say, "This

worked for me, it should work for you". We know that every system functions uniquely. Despite the fact that we have many commonalities, we also have many differences. As in many historical medical philosophies, whether it be homeopathies, Ayurveda or any other modality, we need to address the uniqueness of each body and the disorder itself in order to provide the best healing process.

NINTEEN

Teas

The most famous Western tea for cancer is the Essiac formula. Nurse Caisse (Note: the tea is her name backwards) found that the cure that the North American aboriginals used was this combination of herbs and roots. They pleaded with her not to take it to share it with Western man as they believed it would be destroyed. She did and it was.

What is the famous tea made of?

- Blessed thistle (Cnicus benedictus)
- Burdock root (Arctium lappa)
- Indian rhubarb root (Rheum officinale)
- Red clover (Trifolium pretense)
- Slippery elm inner bark (Ulmus rubra)
- Sheep sorrel (Rumex acetosella)

There is a lot of literature on the Essiac tea and the whole story behind it. To read more, simply go to:

See:
http://campaignfortruth.com/Eclub/250505/ CTM%20-%20story%20of%20essiac.htm

Or you can simply Google, essiac tea.

Coffee

This isn't a section on coffee but if you really want to drink coffee we do have an alternate method for you to make use of it.

The Gerson Institute utilized coffee as an enema. They claimed that the coffee enema was a very powerful, yet safe, means of emptying the bile ducts and thus cleaning out the liver.
As usual, there is a very important caveat: It must only be done when high levels of nutrients and vitamin and mineral replacement are being made. The liver has to be strong and fortified first.

TWENTY

Alkaline water, food, supplements

There are several reasons we want to create an alkaline environment in the body.

1. Cancer thrives in an acidic environment.

2. Cancer even creates an acidic environment.

3. We have over 10,000 enzymes in our bodies. Each group of enzymes works best in a narrow pH range. Most of our enzymes work best in a more alkaline environment.

4. Cancer thrives on glucose, which is acidic, so we want to eliminate sugars from the diet. By eliminating the sugars, we are helping to create an alkaline environment.

5. We also want to reduce meat, poultry and fish. I don't say we have to eliminate them because we need some of the nutrients from them but if we can eat organic, range-fed meat, all the better. In

fact, if you can replace cattle with bison, you are much better off. Eat smaller portions of beef, fewer times during the week. With regard to poultry, again, free-range chicken is a much better choice. Eating fish is a more difficult choice. You want the Omega 3 fatty acids but you have to be careful of the mercury in fish such as salmon and tuna.

6. Water has a better capacity to be anti-oxidant when we eliminate as much of the hydrogen as possible. This, in effect, makes a more alkaline environment.

7. The body thrives with the more alkalizing minerals, for instance, ionic citrate magnesium.

8. There is a lot of information here, and if the body has cancer, we know that the system is already compromised. If the body is compromised, we know that it is not producing the enzymes, transport mechanisms and other components we need to metabolize and absorb a large number of different foods, supplements, tinctures, etc.

It is extremely important to work with a qualified alternative practitioner. Do your research. Understand the kind of cancer you have, the types of treatment (both allopathic and alternative), then decide what is best for you.

Remember, if you decide to deal with your cancer utilizing chemotherapy or radiation, you can still choose a herbal/supplement protocol to protect your body from all the toxicity but you have to know what does and doesn't work with your particular regimen.

TWENTY-ONE

Regardless of where the cancer is...

It is important to realize that wherever the cancer is, you have to look after the liver. Why?

The liver is responsible for other 500 functions. The liver supports every other organ and system in the body. So, regardless of where the cancer is focused or located, we need to protect the liver.

In addition, when looking specifically at liver cancer, Dr. Stanislaw Burzynski's an MD, PhD with a clinic in Houston, Texas, claimed that, "We now know that chemotherapy will speed up the progress of liver cancer. There is no reason to use it. Scientific works have proven beyond any doubt that chemo is completely ineffective, yet doctors are using chemotherapy for liver cancer over and over again. Practically all patients with advanced liver cancer will die." (Suzanne Somers, Knockout)

Dr. Stanislaw Burzynski is known for developing a gene-specific treatment using a combination of cancer-fighting peptides. He has been interviewed by many, including Dr. Mercola, and also has recently released a documentary called, Burzynski, The Movie.

See:
http://www.burzynskimovie.com/

There are many herbs that work for liver health. Chapter 17 details different categories of herbs that operate on the liver in different ways.

TWENTY-TWO

Foods and herbs to protect you from the harms of chemotherapy

Several foods and herbs can help protect the body from the dangers of chemotherapy.

- Liver

- Milk Thistle – to prevent liver inflammation

- See:

  http://www.webmd.com/cancer/news/
  20091214/herb-may-treat-chemotherapy-
  liver-damage

- Essiac tea

Whereas other herbs may interfere with the effectiveness of chemotherapy drugs

Thyroid and Adrenals

The thyroid plays a huge part not only in producing T3 and T4 but also in replenishing red blood cells.

1. Keeping the body warm thus keeping bones warm, and increasing peripheral circulation all help with maintaining red blood cells.

   An easy way to help peripheral blood circulation is to rub cayenne pepper into a small bit of oil and rub into your hands and feet – make sure you rub it off within 15 minutes or you will have burning skin.

   Utilizing the pepper in your cooking will also help.

2. Eliminate the chloride and fluoride from your water. Both are major thyroid suppressants. An easy way to do this is to leave your water on the counter overnight and allow the toxic chemicals to evaporate. Another way is to buy some alkalizing minerals for your water and use the drops in the water before drinking it.

3. We are back to beets again. Not only are they great for the betalaines that fight cancers but they have are great at helping the body build glutathione.

4. In addition, they are well known as a blood purifier and builder.

5. A herb that is great for blood and lymph cleansing and full of nutrients to build

the blood is stinging nettles.

6. Foods like alfalfa are great for their alkaline mineral profile.

7. Take good supplements that have a full spectrum of B vitamins, iron, zinc and copper.

8. Taking thyroid and/or adrenal adaptogens are also enormously beneficial. Gynostemma pentapyllyum is a beautiful adaptogen but there are others like the different ginsengs, gotu kola, rhodiola and licorice.

Red blood cells

Foods that help protect red blood cells are:

- Almonds
- Broccoli (especially the seeds)
- Dried beans and fruits
- Lean red meat (Be careful though. Meat is acidic.)
- Potatoes
- Shellfish
- Tomatoes (Cooked but not canned.)

Herbs that help protect red blood cells are:

- Ashwagandha
- Dandelion

- Parsley
- Red Reishi
- Stinging nettles

White blood cells

Foods that help protect the white blood cells are:

- Green tea

Herbs that help protect the white blood cells are:

- Ashwagandha
- Astragalus
- Cat's claw (but shouldn't be taken if you take insulin for diabetes)
- Red Reishi
- Siberian ginseng

See:
http://www.livestrong.com/article/388428-herbs-to-increase-white-blood-cells/

TWENTY-THREE

Other Modalities

In addition to Western Herbal Medicine, we can look at other modalities. My second Masters Thesis was called, Bridging Ayurvedic, Traditional Chinese Medicine and Western Herbal Medicine. As a result of what I learned, I would be remiss not to mention other cultural modalities. However, one needs to also understand that how they perceive cancer in different cultures is very different as well. The understanding of cancer's evolution, why it happens and how to resolve is all very different from Western understanding.

Ayurvedic

Ayurvedic medicine understands the body in terms of different energetic patterns called Vata, Pitta and Kapha, or movement, transformation and structure.

When these energies are out of balance, imbalance accumulates through the body moving through six stages of dysfunction. Each stage disrupts more variables than the prior one but it is only when we start moving from Stage 5 into Stage 6 that Western allopathic medicine can diagnose or treat symptoms.

Ayurvedic medicine works very differently than allopathic medicine. It does not try to fit everyone into the same box. Instead, it recognizes how unique and individual we each are.

You have to first understand the primary and secondary dosha (energy/metabolic style) of the individual (Vata, Pitta, Kapha) and then understand which pathway the dysfunction took in order to determine what to prescribe.

A good site to give an overall understanding of the various different types of cancers and the protocols utilized is:

See:
http://ayurveda-cancer.org/

German New Medicine

Ryke Geerd Hamer founded German New Medicine in Germany.

He was taken to court and lost his license to practice medicine and his tenure at the university. The claim is that Dr. Hamer presented 6500 cases to court and was able to show a 90% success rate which far outweighs anything chemo, radiation and surgery have ever been able to show. He apparently has investigated and documented over 15,000 cancer cases.

See:
http://customers.hbci.com/~wenonah/new/
hamer.htm

There are 5 basic laws according to German New Medicine:

1. **First rule, or Iron Rule:** Severe diseases originate from shock. The shock's psychological conflict content determines the location of the appearance of a focus in the brain and is called the "Hamer foci".

2. **Second rule:** Two phased nature of disease. If the conflict from the trauma is not resolved, the patient moves into their first active conflict phase.

3. **Third rule:** Ontogenetic system of diseases. Disease progression is controlled by the brain – either the old brain (brain stem and cerebellum) or the new brain (cerebrum).

4. **Fourth rule:** Ontogenetic system of microbes. Microbes do not cause disease but are coordinated by the brain to manage healing processes. Fungi and mycobacterium work with endoderm tissues. Bacteria work with mesoderm tissues. Viruses work with ectoderm tissues.

5. Fifth rule: Healing phase of disease. Created to override daily functions and provide the body the opportunity to focus the healing process.

Thus, according to Hamer, disease does not actually exist. Rather, what allopathic medicine calls disease is actually an effective "special meaningful program of nature" in which fungi, bacteria and virus play a part.

Homeopathic Medicine

Homeopathic medicine is probably the most ecological of all modalities. Ultra-small amounts of a mother tincture are combined with small amounts of water and then shaken in a very specific manner.

Western homeopathy was founded by Dr. Samuel Hahnemans, an MD, who lost faith in Western allopathic medicine. He began to explore different ways to treat people. Allopathic medicine, threatened by his success, or feeling too competitive, set out to prove him wrong by sending one of their best scientific physicians in to work with him. The "spy" was so impressed by Dr. Hahneman's scientific studies and results that he converted.

Western science now finally understands that due to this particular type of movement, the water molecules end up mirroring the tincture. So while the amounts of tincture get smaller and smaller with each combination, the result is actually stronger and stronger. Consequently, despite the fact that old Newtonian chemistry can no longer detect the original mother tincture after a 6x dilution, the remedy actually gets stronger.

Again, the individual makeup is taken into consideration before remedies are determined so you have to work closely with a Homeopathy specialist.

Traditional Chinese Medicine

Chinese Medicine is over 2000 years old. It incorporates a number of components including herbal medicine (the oldest component), acupuncture (12 meridians), massage (Tui na), exercise (Qi Gong) and nutrition.
The theory includes yin/yang, Qi, and the Five Elements. A diagnosis involves an understanding of the characteristics of yin, yang and Qi in terms of:
  • cold and heat
  • inflammation and congestion
  • damp and dry

This chart is taken from Dr. Shen's website and is a great way to summarize some of the Traditional Chinese Herbs used to work with cancer.

See:
http://www.drshen.com/chineseherbsforcanc
er.htm

Some Chinese herbs commonly used to treat cancer:

VITAL-IZE BLOOD AND/OR QI HERBS	ANTI-CANCER HERBS	STRENG THEN-ING HERBS	OTHER HERBS
Chih Ko Aurantium	Rei Shi and various mushrooms	Astragalus Huang Qi	Yi Yi Ren Coix
E Zhu Curcuma Zedoaria	Lu Feng Fan Hornet Nest	Xi Yang She American Ginseng	LuGen Phragmites
Tao Ren Persicae Semen	Long Kui Solanum	Shu Di Hua Chinese Foxglove Root	Bai Mao G Imperata
Hong Hua Carthami Tinctori	Ban Zhi Liar Scutellaria	Gan Cao Chinese Licorice Root	Mu Li - Oy Shell and other shells
San Leng Sparganii Rhizoma	Dong Ling C Rabdosime Rubescentis	Dang Gui Angelica Sinensis	Pu Gong Y Taraxacum
Wu Ling Sh Trogoptero ri Pteromi	Bai Hua She Cao Oldenlandia	Bie Jia Turtle shell	Ji Xue Ten Millettia

---

The Gerson Program

Dr. Max Gerson was one of the first medical physicians who worked with a nutritional metabolic program.

Similar to Dr. Hamer, his records reveal that his patients recovered well and they lived long healthy lives. He worked with various celebrities including Albert Schweitzer who claimed Gerson was "one of the most eminent medical geniuses in the history of medicine." (How to Fight Cancer and Win, 2000, p. 311).

However, unlike Dr. Hamer, Dr. Gerson believed that the following contributed to the evolution cancer:

- Compromised liver
- Compromised pancreas
- Poor nutrition
- Exposure to herbicides, pesticides, fertilizers
- Immune system breakdown

Similar to Dr. Hamer, he believed that you don't just treat the localized cancer but rather the whole body and the whole person.

Two major components of the Gerson program are:

- Detoxification
- Nutritional replacement

(Detoxification and nutritional replacement are the basis of all the medicinal theories throughout history. However, these practices are missing in today's conventional medicine despite that we require them more than ever.)

In order to support the whole body, the program provides a diet rich in whole natural foods, like:

- Grains
- Vegetables
- Fruits

All organic foods with no additives and no:

- Sugar
- White flour
- Coffee

The body is strengthened with additional:

- Vitamins
- Minerals
- Enzymes

Hyperthermia

Hyperthermia is a method that provokes a high alkalinity by increasing the body's temperature. Again, it has been utilized throughout history in various cultures.

The program starts with providing the body with a tremendous amount of nutrients using foods, herbs and supplements.

It then provokes the body into a fever sweat using either herbs or technology. The duration of the fever correlates with the extensiveness of the cancer.

The therapy provokes an increase in white blood cells in the immune system. These white blood cells in turn fight off the cancer. Both the heat and the alkalinity are thought to address the cancer cells.

Even the U.S. National Cancer Institute acknowledged that heat therapy increases the effectiveness of other treatments to the point of 25 - 35%, in 1989. (Fischer, How to Fight Cancer and Win, 2000, p. 319)

TWENTY-FOUR

What to avoid and what to eat

The following is a simple guide for healthy eating.

AVOID	TAKE
microwaved foods	slightly steamed foods
barbecued foods	foods cooked at a low temperature
processed foods, oils,	honey, coconut oil
sugar, high fructose corn syrup, aspartame & other artificial sugars	
GMO foods: soybean, corn,	real foods
Margarine, hydrogenated oils	butter
Foods with preservatives, artificial/natural flavorings, MSG	whole fresh foods
Table salt (has sodium, chloride, & aluminum)	sea salt or mineral salt

sodium nitrites	baking soda
sodium benzoates	garlic
bottled water	alkalized water
alcohol	herbal teas, green tea
sodas or soft drinks	homemade juice without added sugar

TWENTY-FIVE

What to do now

There is always a variety of variables to take into consideration when healing the body. This is your body. Take responsibility and do your own research. (You have obviously already started so, congratulations).

It is also important to find a health practitioner in whom you have faith. Look for a practitioner with whom you feel a connection, someone who listens to you, works with you and deals effectively and honestly with all of your questions and concerns. Working with a practitioner who can help you organize your thoughts, will support your emotions and will be your healing advocate is vital.

Know what you want from your health practitioner. Do you want?

- Someone who deals with the facts without emotion?
- Someone who connects with what you are going through emotionally?
- Someone who will make all decisions

for you?

- Someone who will support the decisions you want to make?

- Someone who deals with the conventional?

- Someone who works with leading edge therapies?

- Someone who integrates nutrition, herbs, and other modalities?

- Someone who knows what conventional treatments to provide and doesn't deal with anything else?

I recommend that you always get a second opinion. Theoretically, factors that can impact on a given physician's opinions are:

- Technology available
- School of thought
- Individual methods of treatment
- Experience with the given diagnosis.

While second opinions may be awkward for the doctor and patient at times, studies have shown that 30 percent of patients who sought second opinions for elective surgery and 18 percent of those who were required to obtain a second opinion by their insurance company found that the two opinions were not in agreement.

These studies reinforce why you need to make sure you are educated properly to make the best decision for your health.

See: http://www.patientadvocate.org/index.php?p=691

Unfortunately, in allopathic medicine, you often find that additional opinions will simply support the first. No one wants to take responsibility for saying something different. So make sure that whoever you see answers your questions.

Know your rights:

- You always have the right to a second opinion.

- You may not have the right to choose what kind of treatment you want, even if it is your own body.

- You may not have the right to choose what kind of treatment to engage in if it is your child.

TWENTY-SIX

Some closing thoughts

Look at your diagnosis as an opportunity to reach your greatest potential. Embrace your journey of healing with gratitude and appreciation that you have the opportunity to take a break from the outside world, to grow and learn within.

Recognize your mind as your greatest resource. Do your research. Maximize the "placebo effect" and make it work for you. Stay calm, stay focused, and know that your body was designed with phenomenal healing capacity. Surround yourself with others who are connected to your healing journey.

And remember, how you do the journey is more important than the end result. So embrace it for all it's worth.

APPENDIX 1

Further Reading

Mark Duxbury and Dean McClennan, former sales reps for Johnson & Johnson, claim that "their careers at Johnson & Johnson's Ortho Biotech unit were based mostly on lies", and that "the bulk of their business selling Procrit to hospitals and clinics was conducting Medicare fraud."

See:
http://www.cbsnews.com/8301-505123_162-42842558/drug-rep-in-3b-procrit-case-80-of-my-sales-were-medicare-fraud-carried-400k-in-cash/

Big Pharma behind war?

See:
http://www.naturalnews.com/036339_pearl_harbor_big_pharma_ig_farben.html

For other Venn diagrams showing the cross over management of the US Senate:

http://EndtheLie.com/2012/04/18/18-venn-diagrams-showing-how-corrupted-american-

---

democracy-really-is/#ixzz1zVHv8hcg

Famous Quotes about Cancer:

http://www.globalhealingcenter.com/truth-
about-cancer/chemotherapy-quotes

To find a list of drugs and what nutrients they
deplete, go to www.choicesunlimited.ca/

Alternative treatments and statistics, go to:

http://www.cancertutor.com/
http://www.anoasisofhealing.com/
http://articles.mercola.com/sites/articles/arc
hive/2011/04/23/dr-nicholas-gonzalez-on-
alternative-cancer-treatments.aspx
http://www.alternative-cancer-care.com/
http://www.burzynskiclinic.com/

APPENDIX II

A brief story

The article below discusses someone else look-ing for statistics on cancer. He wrote that he could not find the statistics because:

• The author was concerned about coming un-der the full hammer of the Food and Drug Administration (FDA).

• That's like going to war with the United States, trying to stay "under the radar" of the FDA. The authors are just a small operation trying to help people.

• Is there any wonder why these small clinics don't publish their statistics? Answer: No, they don't want the hassles and lawsuits.

So, What Did I Find?

• On our first meeting, I asked my clinic doctor about his statistics.

• He told me he had been tracking over 400 of his cancer patients who used Alternative Can-cer Treatments for more than four years on various Types of Cancer.

He said the group had an amazing 85% success

story, meaning 85% of his tracked cancer patients were either in remission, or their cancer was completely gone. I sat there truly amazed as I listened to his story of success with Alternative Cancer Treatments.

• Important Note: These are cancer victims usually in stage 3 and 4 where it has spread to other organs and tissues of the body. These are difficult cases for traditional cancer treatments and their 5-year survival rates are usually in single digits.

• And most, if not all, of these cancer victims have already tried traditional treatments and they failed.

See:
http://www.cancer-research-awareness.com/alternative-cancer-treatment-st...

APPENDIX III

Chocolate is an incredibly nutrient dense food. Like most fruits and vegetables, the majority of nutrient is condensed in the seed.

The seed of cocoa fruit has over 1200 molecules and over 300 nutrients in the seed, in significant amounts, that are beneficial to the body.

There are 1000s of known anti-oxidants. Some are stronger than others; each works in differently locations, i.e., inside the cell, the cell membrane, and outside of the cell. Further different ones work on different types of free radicals. Finally some are weak and some are strong.

In chocolate we have two predominant categories of epicatechins and procynandins, which are not only very powerful anti-oxidants but they are found in huge amounts.

Together these types of bioflavonoids have a variety of effects on cancer cells:

1) They turn on apoptosis (cell death) in cancer cells
2) They alter the cell membrane of cancer

cells letting in oxygen instead of glucose thus changing the environment from acidic to alkaline

3) They block angiogenesis (creation of new blood vessels to bring in more nutrients to the tumor.

In addition, good Xocai™ chocolate has a good load of alkalizing minerals and lots of other nutrients the body needs.

It could be argued that the cancer cells also need these nutrients, which is true BUT good chocolate is also turning on cell death and blocking the nutrients from getting into the cancer cells…so guess who benefits from the nutrients?

My book, *The Chocolate Controversy: Tthe bad, the mediocre and the awesome* – goes into much more detail.

APPENDIX IV

Herbs and Foods that block angiogenesis:

1. Chocolate, green tea – contain polyphenols called "catechins" or epigallocatechin gallate (EGCG). The EGCG blocks receptors on a cells surface that issue command for the creation of new blood vessels.

2. Red wine – "resveratrol" – while there are a number of claims about resveratrol, what people don't broadcast is that you need pepperine molcules to absorb that anti-oxidant AND it is only available in good organic wines. (this is not an endorsement to drink, quantities of >100ml per day seem to lose their protective effect). Finally, Professor Riboli of the famous EPIC study thinks this study was poorly designed and conclusions are questionable.

3. garli – "dialyl sulphide"

4. cabbage, kale, brussels sprouts – cruciferous vegetables contain "indol-3-carbinol"

5. rosemary – "carnosol"

6. raspberries, strawberries, walnuts, hazel nuts and pecan – contain polyphenol called "ellagic acid". Ellagic acid has been demonstrated to act against 2 most common mechanisms of stimulation of blood vessels: VEGF and PDGF.

7. mushrooms – shiitake, maitake, kawaratake, enokitake contain "lentinan" and other polysaccharides

8. broccoli – "sulphoraphane"

9. turmeric – "curcumin", a yellow powder used in Indian curries. Also, one of the most potent naturally occurring anti-inflammatory agents. In the laboratory it has been shown to inhibit angiogenesis and promote cancer cells death or cell "apoptosis". Indians have less than 20% of colon, breast, lung and kidney cancers compared to Westerners of the same age. This is true despite high exposure to environmental toxins on a worse scale than in the West. Could their diet have something to do with the favourable statistics?

10. tomatoes – "lycopene"

11. soy beans – "genistein", "daidzein" and "glyciteine". Researchers wrote that "soy and green tea may be used as potentially effective dietary regimen for inhibiting progression of oestrogen-dependent breast cancer". Soy phyto-oestrogens act along similar lines as common breast cancer drug Tamoxifen.

12. ginger – "6 -gingerol"

13. cherries – "glucaric acid" which can facilitate elimination of xenoestrogens from environmental chemicals

14. blueberries, cranberries, cinnamon, dark chocolate – "anthocyanidins" and "proanthocyanidins"

15. parsley and celery – "apigenine"

16. rosemary, thyme, oregano, basil and mint – essential oils of the terpene family

17. seaweed – "fucoidan" and "fucoxanthin"

18. salmon, tuna, trout, meckarel, cod, sardine – omega-3s

19. orange, mandarin, lemon, grapefruit – anti-inflammatory 'flavinoids'

20. pomegranate – antioxidant

21. yoghurt – 'probiotics'

22. vitamin D

23. selenium

If taking chemotherapy then the following needs to be addressed:

1. Pomegranate: should NOT be taken with chemo; as the CYP3A4 liver enzyme that metabolizes most drugs is deactivated by pomegranate; 96.8% blockage of midazolam 1'-hydroxylation

2. Star fruit: 99.9% blockage of midazolam 1'-hydroxylation

3.Pawpaw: blocks 88% of midazolam 1'- hydroxylation

4. Grapefruit: blocks 85% of midazolam 1'-hydroxylation

So you have to be careful with these fruits – either you eat the fruit OR you take the chemo – NOT both.

Another good source of information regarding herb reactions with cancer medications is Sloan Kettering

See:
http://www.mskcc.org/mskcc/html/11570.cf
m

I love this website:
http://www.eattodefeat.org/food

Dr. Pack's summary on Natural Angiogenesis Inhibitors and Cancer is also good:

http://www.rainbow.coop/index.php?src=dir
ecto-
ry&view=nutritional_library&srctype=detail&r
efno=3693&submenu=NutritionalLibrary

Also, if food can inhibit than food should also be able to promote angiogenesis. The following website provides some good information/ studies on various foods that can either promote or inhibit angiogenesis.

References:

Posted necessary references throughout book for your convenience.

Books & Journals & Institutes

Department of Chemistry, Simon Fraser University, Burnaby, BC, V5A 1S6, Canada

Baylock, Russell, MD. Health and Nutrition Secrets. Health Press, NA, 2006.

Baylock, Russell, MD. Excitotoxins: The taste that Kills. Health Press, NA, 1996.

Fischer, William L. How to Fight Cancer & Win. Agora South, Baltimore, Maryland, 2000.

German Cancer Research Center, Pharmaceutical Biology (C015), Im Neuenheimer Feld 280, 69120 Heidelberg, Germany

Institute of Toxicology, University of Mainz, Obere Zahlbacher Straße 67, 55131 Mainz, Germany, Available online 17 July 2007.

Tanton, David. Taking the Mystery Out of Cancer. Cancer Prevention and Cure is Possible. Soaring Heights Publishing, Springfield, OR, 2011.

Weil, Andrew, MD. 8 weeks to Optimal Health. Ballantin Books, NY, 1998.

Baselt, R.. Disposition of Toxic Drugs and Chemicals in Man, 8th edition, Biomedical Publications, Foster City, CA, 2008, pp. 547-549.

Edwards, Jim (August 17, 2009), Drug Rep in $3B Procrit Case: "80% of My Sales Were Medicare Fraud"; Carried $400K in "Cash"

See:
http://www.cbsnews.com/8301-505123_162-
42842558/drug-rep-in-3b-procrit-case-80-of-
my-sales-were-medicare-fraud-carried-400k-in-
cash/

Engelberg, Alfred B. et al. *Balancing innovation,
access, and profits -- marketing exclusivity for biologics*, N Engl J Med 361:1917

Hardell L, Walker MJ, Walhjalt B, Friedman
LS, Richter ED (March 2007). *"Secret ties to in-
dustry and conflicting interests in cancer research"*.
Am. J. Ind. Med. 50 (3): 227–33.

Napoli, Maryann (October 5, 2011), Whistle-
blower's story: New book reviewed, Center for
MedicalConsumers.

See:
http://medicalconsumers.org/2011/10/05/w
histleblowers-story-new-book-reviewed/

Walsh, G, Spada, S. "Epogen/Procrit" in: Direc-
tory of approved biopharmaceutical products.
CRC Press, 2005, pp.39-41.

Vimala, S., et al. *Anti-tumour promoter activity in
Malaysian ginger rhizobia used in traditional medicine*. British Journal of Cancer, Vol. 80, No. 1/2,

April 1999, pp. 110-16

Andreas Gescher, Ugo Pastorino, Simon M Plummer, Margaret M Manson. *Suppression of tumour development by substances derived from the diet – mechanisms and clinical implications.* Br J Clin Pharmacol. 1998 January; 45(1): 1–12.

Iqbal M, et al. Pharmacol Toxicol. 2003 Jan, 92(1):33-8

- Agaricus Blazei Murrill. 1970
- Am Heart Journal 06; 252(6): 1028-1034
- Ausubel, Kenny. When Healing Becomes a Crime. Healing Arts Press, Rochester, Vermont, 2000.
- Campbell, Colin. The China Study. 2004
- Dr. D Gary Young, Essential Oils Desk Reference, 2002
- Fischer, William L. How to Fight Cancer and Win, 2000.
- Indian Journal of Physiology and Pharmacology, 2001, Vol. 45, Issue 2, pp. 253-257
- Somers, Suzanne. Knock Out. Three Rivers Press, 2009
- Tanton, David. Taking the Mystery Out of Cancer. 2011

Trudeau, Kevin. Natural Cures. Alliance Publishing Group, Inc., Elk Grove Village, IL, 2005.

(controversial)

Dr. Burzynski is just one of the alternative cancer specialists. There are many others as well,
such as the Gerson Therapy and Dr. Nick Gonzalez's nutritional approach – or even medical
marijuana. Unfortunately, the system as currently configured is stacked against you receiving these potentially life-saving therapies (and
others like them).

Knowledge is always one of the highest forms of
power so I also recommend you share this information with your friends and loved ones. The
film, Cut Poison Burn which documents the Navarros' story, is an easy and powerful way to do
so and is being sold on a "value-priced" basis to
help the Navarros' pay off Thomas' medical bills.
This means that you can download a copy of the
film for $1.99 and up; depending on how much
you're willing to pay. You can also purchase a
DVD copy for $9.99.

A percentage of the proceeds from the film will go
to cancer organizations that donate 100 percent of
their proceeds to families fighting cancer, not to
the American Cancer Society. I am also making
the DVD available on my website. Of these proceeds, 80 percent will go to the producers and Jim
Navarro's family. I'm giving the remaining 20 percent to the Grassroots Health's Breast Cancer Prevention Project. All monies donated from the sale

of Cut Poison Burn will be used to enroll women aged 60 and over in a project aimed to demonstrate the effectiveness of Vitamin D in breast cancer prevention. More information about this project can be found at:

http://www.grassrootshealth.net/press-20110805

Videos to watch:

http://www.youtube.com/watch?v=hQicB_7KNL8

http://www.youtube.com/watch?v=gWLrfNJICeM&feature=related

Websites to search:

www.choicesunlimited.ca
www.healthiertalk.com

Dr. W.C. Douglass   www.healthiertalk.com
Dr. Mark Hyman   www.drhyman.com
Dr. Mercola   www.mercola.com

Dr. Al Sears
    www.healthiertalk.com
Dr. David Tanton   www.drtanto.com

Dr. Julian Whitaker
    www.youtube.com/watch?v=kxLSUaKb4pI

Jenny Thompson   www.hsionline.com

Jon Christian Ryter
    http://www.jonchristianryter.com/

Kevin Trudeau
    www.ktradionetwork.com
http://www.forhealthfreedom.org/Publicatio
ns/Monopoly/wsj-970602.html
www.cancerinform.org/kids1.html
www.naturalnews.com

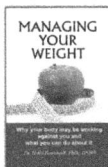

Managing Your Weight
Why your body may be working against you and what you can do about it.

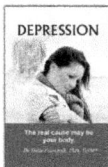

Depression
The real cause may be your body

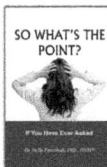

So What's the Point
If you have ever asked

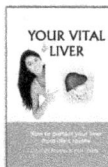

Your Vital Liver
How to protect your liver from life's toxins

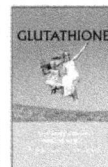

Glutathione
Your body's secret healing agent

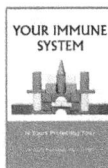

Your Immune System
Is yours protecting you?

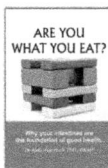

Are You What You Eat?
Why your intestines are the foundation of good health.

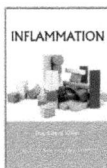

Inflammation
The Silent Killer

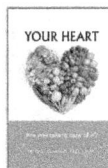

Your Heart
Are you taking care of it?

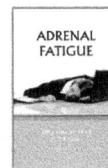

Adrenal Fatigue
Why am I so tired all the time?

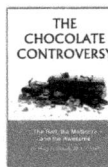

The Chocolate Controversy
The Bad, the Mediocre and the Awesome

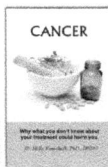

Cancer
Why what you don't know about your treatment could harm you.

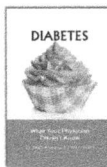

Diabetes
What your physician doesn't know

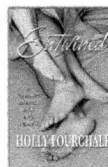

Entwined
A Romantic Journey back into Health